Victim of Love?

HOW YOU CAN BREAK THE CYCLE OF BAD RELATIONSHIPS

TOM WHITEMAN, PH.D.
AND RANDY PETERSEN

 PIÑON PRESS

P.O. Box 35007, Colorado Springs, Colorado 80935

Library of Congress Catalog Card Number: 98-12182

ISBN 1-57683-053-5

Photo by Superstock

Some of the anecdotal illustrations in this book are true to life and are included with the permission of the persons involved. All other illustrations are composites of real situations, and any resemblance to people living or dead is coincidental.

"ADDICTED TO LOVE" was written by Robert Palmer. Copyright © 1985 Bungalow Music N.V. Used by permission. All rights reserved.

Unless otherwise identified, all Scripture quotations in this publication are taken from the *HOLY BIBLE: NEW INTERNATIONAL VERSION* ® (NIV®). Copyright © 1973, 1978, 1984 by International Bible Society. Used by permission of Zondervan Publishing House. All rights reserved.

Whiteman, Tom.
    Victim of love? : how you can break the cycle of a bad relationship (and get on with your life) / Thomas Whiteman, Randy Petersen.
        p.   cm.
    ISBN 1-57683-053-5 (pbk.)
    1. Relationship addiction—Popular works.   2. Relationship addiction—Case studies.   3.   Sex addiction—Case studies.   4. Obsessive-compulsive disorder—Case studies. I. Petersen, Randy. II. Title.
RC552.R44W47 1989
616.86—dc21   98-12182
                                                                                      CIP

Printed in the United States of America

1 2 3 4 5 6 7 8 9 10 11 12 13 14 15 / 99 98

Contents

Introduction   5
Chapter One: The Circle   9
Chapter Two: Types of Addictive Relationships   23
Chapter Three: Case Study: Sally   37
Chapter Four: Characteristics of Addictive Relationships   45
Chapter Five: Test Yourself   71
Chapter Six: Case Study: Scott   79
Chapter Seven: The Roots of Addiction   89
Chapter Eight: Case Study: Bonnie   103
Chapter Nine: Breaking the Addictive Cycle   113
Chapter Ten: The Slope   129
Chapter Eleven: Case Study: Laurie   155
Chapter Twelve: Best Friends   163
Chapter Thirteen: Balance   173
Chapter Fourteen: Boundaries   181
Chapter Fifteen: Case Study: Christine   191
Chapter Sixteen: Addiction Within a Marriage   199
Chapter Seventeen: Addiction in a Same-sex Friendship   215
Chapter Eighteen: Family Relationships   221
Chapter Nineteen: Conclusion   229
Notes   233
About the Authors   235

Introduction

WHY WOULD AN INTELLIGENT WOMAN STAY WITH A MAN WHO ABUSES her? Why do so many competent single women seem to settle for men who appear to be so "beneath" them?

How can a man who has everything going for him—a good job, a fine home, a loving wife and children—have an affair that could jeopardize everything?

Why does a parent—whose job it is to prepare a child for life outside the home—continue to "baby" a child well into adulthood and restrict that child's development as an independent person?

These may all be examples of addictive relationships, relationships driven by a compulsive urge rather than sacrificial love.

Is this just the latest entry in the Addiction-of-the Month Club? Talk shows are booked solid with workaholics, spendaholics, food addicts, gambling addicts, and TV addicts. Are we merely inventing another excuse for another weakness—love addiction?

I don't think so. I believe that millions of individuals are walking around with addictive personalities, though they have never used drugs or been drunk. Instead, these people act out their addictive tendencies in ways that are more socially acceptable. And what could be more acceptable than love? These people crave a fix from their lovers or fantasies, just as surely as any junkie craves a fix from drugs.

Have you ever said or thought the following?

"I'll just die if I can't be with him."

"If she leaves me I'll do something drastic."

"You're my everything. I'd be nothing without you."

While these words make for nice poetry—or even hit love songs—in reality they smack of a relationship that's way out of balance. Don't worry; if you've said such things, it doesn't prove you're in an addictive relationship, but you may want to investigate further just how dependent you are.

Don't get me wrong. This book is not anti-relationship. Healthy relationships are one of the best things in life—they're healing, restorative, pleasurable. But unhealthy relationships are disastrous. This book will help you identify danger signs, avoid or escape from bad relationships, and establish healthy relationship habits.

Many people I deal with in my counseling practice are single—divorced or never married. As a result, many of my examples have to do with romantic addictions in dating relationships. But unhealthy addictions also can occur in the context of marriage, so I've included a special chapter for that situation because slightly different rules apply. Same-sex friendships and family relationships also can be troubled by addictive tendencies. Other chapters will focus on these areas.

No matter what your specific situation is, most of the general principles of addictive relationships—how you got in and how to get out—will pertain to you. And that's the focus of the bulk of this book.

I first became aware of addictive relationships about ten years ago as a counselor at Life Counseling Services in Paoli, Pennsylvania. I would frequently encounter clients, usually women, who seemed to be making some very poor choices in relationships. What confused me was that even when these clients knew what to look for in a relationship, and even when they were determined to hold out for a healthy partner, inevitably they would repeat the same mistake by choosing another person who was all wrong for them.

I was frustrated. Week after week we'd go over the same principles, and each week they seemed even more determined to break off their addictive relationship. But somehow they were never able to overcome the compelling lure of the other person. I gradually concluded that sheer willpower was not enough. I was struck by the similarities between these people and drug addicts I had observed. Relationships were, for these women, their drug of choice. I had observed the difficulties that substance abusers faced. Even when they knew that drug or alcohol use was tearing them apart, they seemed unable to overcome its viselike grip on their life. The most effective method I found for overcoming these addictions was through a "cold turkey" inpatient treatment program, followed by close accountability through a support group or sponsor.

When I heard these women talk about their destructive relationships and their inability to overcome the hold of another person on their lives, I wondered if they needed similar treatment. We could not provide a thirty-day treatment program or a detox unit, but I was able to put together a support group of seven clients who were all struggling with seemingly similar problems. The Group, as we called it, decided to meet two nights a week because they all felt that they needed close accountability and support.

There was one problem. What materials would this group use? What treatment method would work with a group like this? I didn't know of any materials available for these specific needs, so I decided to adapt some material developed for those recovering from other kinds of addictions. Although much of the group was educational in nature, there was also great benefit from our shared stories and the loving accountability that we brought each other from week to week.

This first support group served as the foundation for much of the material presented in this book, which has been supplemented over the years by seminars, additional support groups, and counseling with many other individuals. I acknowledge their courage and determination in sharing their stories and am grateful that they decided to step forward and begin talking about the struggle and guilt they've faced in these difficult relationships.

The five case studies appear with the consent of the people involved. I've changed all the names and some of the details of the stories to protect people's identities. As you read about The Group, be aware that you're seeing the other characters in these people's lives through their lenses, which are biased. In truth, the others may not be as bad as they seem from these stories. There is always another side to every story.

Other stories appear from time to time in the text. I've struggled to maintain both the confidentiality of the counseling office and my journalistic integrity. In some cases, I've developed composite characters, mixtures of various people I've known or counseled. The mixing of details will certainly make these people unrecognizable and thus preserve their privacy. However, the essential facts and the lessons learned are accurate.

As you read the struggles of the men and women who contributed their stories to this book, I hope they will enlighten and inspire you. If you are suffering in an addictive relationship, these pages may give you the push you need to take a first step or two toward health.

CHAPTER ONE

The Circle

℘

I T'S A HOT AND STICKY JULY NIGHT. SEVEN PEOPLE SIT IN A CIRCLE OF chairs in my counseling office. There's some small talk while everyone arrives, but now that everyone's here it's silent.

There is an awkwardness here, as heavy as the muggy air. I try to ease things with a friendly introduction. "You may wonder why I've called you here tonight. You don't know each other— yet. But each of you has spent some time talking with me about difficult situations you're facing. As you'll soon see, some of your situations are amazingly similar. I thought it would be helpful to compare notes."

I don't want to force anyone to speak up, so I ask for a volunteer to go first. The silence returns. No one looks me in the eye. Then Dawn, perhaps because she's sitting next to me, clears her throat softly, takes a deep breath, and speaks.

"I got divorced about five years ago. Maybe I'm still not over it. Since then, I've been in four relationships. I guess you'd call them intimate relationships. It's hard for me to admit that, because I . . . well, I really don't believe in being like that. But it's been really hard."

Dawn takes another deep breath and continues. "Right now

I'm seeing a man. I care a lot about him. But I'm not sure what he thinks of me. He's married."

I begin to ask some questions, gently guiding Dawn through her story. She grew up with an alcoholic father and remembers deep longings for his unhindered affection. She married young, but that relationship soured soon after the honeymoon. She tried hard to make it work, "but apparently not hard enough," she sighs.

The divorce was his idea, a rejection that wounded her deeply. She sought healing in the arms of other men, landing in one unhealthy romance after another. She describes a chain of emotionally abusive—sometimes physically abusive—relationships. Yet she remained faithful in each one. The men "tired" of her, she explains. "I don't know what's wrong with me," she says coldly, "but it didn't take any of them very long to find out."

Like several of the other group members, Dawn was raised in a religious home. It was a rocky road for her. Each new relationship began with a solid conviction about sexual restraint, but in the heat of passion and the fire of self-doubt, those convictions melted. Dawn hated herself for giving in so easily, but tried to justify it in various ways. After all, since her divorce she was "damaged goods." And she would never get the love she needed from men without giving something in return.

And now there was this married man. "I just like being with him," she says. "He made me feel special. At first I thought it could just be a strong friendship. Whatever else I was, I was not a *homewrecker*. Well, I guess I didn't have to worry about that because there is no way he is going to leave his wife for me. I'm just a side dish. But it got romantic and physical, and I'm in so deep that now I can't get out. I must admit, there's something exciting about it. Something bad. I hate it and I love it at the same time." Dawn glances over at me, seeking approval and fearing judgment.

"I know I have to stop seeing him," she says slowly, articulating each word. "I know that. But he's inside of me. I *need* him."

As I look around the circle, I see some nods of encouragement. These people know what she's talking about. They've been there. Some, though, are still staring at the floor. Maybe Dawn's story hit too close to home.

"Thank you," I say to Dawn. "And thank you for having the guts to speak first. It's not easy, I know. I'm wondering if we can just go around the circle. Margie, would you like to tell us about your situation?"

Margie is in her mid-twenties, pretty and energetic. "I was hoping you'd go the other direction," she says wryly, then a smile crosses her face. "But, okay, I'll go. What do you want to know?"

"Why are you here?"

"Because my boyfriend's busy tonight." Margie's face is like the sky on a partly cloudy day. Her natural energy normally radiates through her facial expressions, but then a cloud passes, and all turns dark. "That's really true," she adds, with a dark cynicism. "And that's really why I'm here."

Margie described her boyfriend as "a ladies' man." He treats her like a princess, but she wonders how many other princesses are in his court. They've never been able to talk about this because "I'm afraid of saying something dumb and losing him," she says. "Whenever we talk about anything even remotely resembling commitment or the future or—God forbid—marriage, he clams up or changes the subject, and then I don't see him for a week."

There are mumbles of recognition from the other women in the circle. They know those symptoms.

I ask Margie about her upbringing. She grew up without a father in her home and was probably overly dependent on her mother. She dated a lot as a teenager and into her twenties, but found that several steady relationships quickly went way out of balance. "I needed the guy more than he needed me," she says. "That always causes problems. And I guess now it's the same old story."

Her sunny look comes out again, briefly. "In a lot of ways I'm lucky, I guess. My boyfriend is a really great guy. He takes me to very expensive restaurants and exciting places. Believe me, I've dated a lot of toads whose idea of a night on the town is a hockey game and a few beers afterward. I should count my blessings." Then the clouds roll in. "But lots of times he is mysteriously unavailable. Some weekends, he's just gone. No explanation. I keep hoping he's an international spy or something, but I know he's got to be seeing someone else. I called his answering machine thirty times one weekend. That's all I did. I sat at home and moped and punched the buttons on the phone. I know I should stand up for my rights, be strong. But I'm really afraid he'll go. And what will I do then? I figure a nice date once in a while is better than no date at all."

Joy speaks next. She proudly proclaims to the group that she has had only one true love in her whole life. She starting dating her husband in ninth grade and finally married him while they were in college. They have been married now for about fourteen years. "And now," Joy says, her voice cracking, "we're separated."

There are a few empathetic moans from the group. Dawn digs out a tissue from her purse and offers it to Joy, who just clutches it in her hand.

"My husband has wanted a divorce for about three years now," Joy continues, "but I've said no. Maybe I'm crazy, but I just believe that God will bring him back to me. I still love him, in spite of everything, and I don't see how he can walk away from that. And we have three children." Young children. Joy is barely thirty herself. As Joy speaks of the difficulty of raising the kids on her own, her anger shows. She is normally mild-mannered, but there is a fury raging inside her. "My husband is currently living with someone else, and he says he's giving me all the child-support money he can afford, but I know he's spending a lot on her. That really bothers me. I mean, where is his responsibility? It's with me. And the children. Not with her."

"If it hurts so much," asks Dawn, "why don't you just let him go?" It's not an attack, just a question. And as soon as she asks it,

Dawn knows there's no good answer. *Why don't you just let him go?* Each woman in the group wrestles with that issue. It's far easier to say it than to do it.

"Lots of my friends ask me that," Joy responds. "They say I should move on with my life, get the divorce. But I love him. Don't you see? There are vows there, promises we have made to each other. He may break his word, but that doesn't mean I can break mine. I believe in the power of love. I believe in the power of God. I must remain faithful. I don't know what God is doing here, to test me or what, but I have to keep loving my husband. I still believe that someday he will see the error of his ways and come back."

After a few moments of silence, all eyes turn to Laurie, next in line. She is about forty, impeccably made up and dressed to kill. Come to think of it, I have never seen her in anything less than the height of business fashion. She seems the essence of the assertive modern woman.

"Never date anyone you work with," she says boldly. "Never. Never. Never."

"Is that the voice of experience?" Margie quips.

Laurie looks over to her and nods slowly. "I'm here because I broke my own rule. I knew better. Eight months ago, my boss started coming on to me, and I should have given him a stop sign right away. But I kind of liked the attention. And he paid a *lot* of attention to me—seven hours a day, five days a week. Maybe he wore me down, I don't know. But we started dating, casually at first. Then not so casually."

The relationship is bad, Laurie says, and she knows she needs to get out of it. But she doesn't know how. "He's a really sexy guy, but he's a real jerk, too. I don't know why those two qualities go together so very often, but this guy's at the top of the list in both categories." She details how he takes advantage of her in the office and in private. He pushed her to surrender to him sexually in ways she never intended and uses her devotion to help himself professionally. Laurie feels miserable and trapped.

"Every day I think, Okay, this is the day it ends. But then I see him and lose my nerve. He has this power over me. I don't know how to say it. I want him. I want to be with him all the time." Laurie admits to the group that she's divorced and has no desire to marry again. "I swore I would never again let a man have that kind of power over me," she states. "But here I am, unable or unwilling to get this man out of my life, out of my heart, even though I know it's all wrong."

David is the only man in the group other than me. With a flippant comment about "equal time," I invite him to speak. I assume he must feel some discomfort at the male bashing that's gone on so far, but he shows no sign of hesitancy.

"I guess I'm the guy you're all talking about," he smiles. "The jerk, the ladies' man, the one who takes advantage. Are men really that bad?"

"They're worse," says Laurie.

"Yeah," Margie adds. "You should hear what we'd say if you guys weren't here!"

A tension-easing laughter fills the room. This is good. The group is working as it should. The initial awkwardness has worn off. Some therapeutic connections are being made.

"Seriously," David resumes, "I am like that, like those other guys, though I'm not proud to admit it. And I guess in some ways I'm like you. Maybe it will help to get a male perspective."

"Fire away," I say.

"I'm in my thirties and single—never married. That means I've had a lot of years of dating. I'd say there have been nine or ten pretty intense relationships—steady relationships—in that time, and a handful of minor ones. Most of them fit the same pattern."

David goes on to say how it started with his first girlfriend, back in high school. He worshipped her from afar for over a year, until finally she returned his interest and they began dating. The reality didn't match the fantasy. After a few months he broke up with her.

David's face shows pain even now as he retells it. "I hated doing that. She was a great person, but I just didn't want her anymore. That sounds cruel, doesn't it? But it's the truth. And I've done the same thing again and again. I idolize a woman, a relationship starts, and I'm disappointed that she's not the perfect woman I wanted."

"But no one's perfect," says Dawn.

"I know," David replies. "And maybe I don't mean exactly perfect but *perfectly fulfilling for me*. You know? I'm looking for a woman who will be right for me, someone who will strengthen my strengths and make up for my failings. She doesn't need to be perfect, but she needs to be *right* for me."

David rehearses the pattern of intense pursuit, euphoric conquest, and ultimate disillusionment. He obviously regrets the pain he has caused along the way, but explains, "That's the way I am. I have high standards."

As I prod him for details, he reveals that his standards are astronomical—looks, intelligence, humor, spirituality, creativity. "The Bionic Woman," Margie jokes.

What's more, David says he feels an emptiness that he expects this wonder woman to fill. "I keep looking, all the time," he says. "It's like my major goal in life, to find the right woman and love her like crazy. Every time I walk into a room, I think maybe *she* will be there. I know that's corny, but I'm always checking out every woman I see. Will she measure up? Will she be *the one?*"

"What about *this* room?" asks Laurie, sitting beside him. "Have you been 'checking us out'?"

David looks suddenly shy, his eyes darting along the floor. "Well, to be honest, yes."

I seize the moment. "That's honest. Thanks, David. Remember, we're not here to judge each other. We're here to share our situations, to compare notes. And I believe we're up to Ginnie."

Ginnie is the most soft-spoken person in the group. There is a deep beauty in her dark eyes, but she has done nothing to draw attention to it. She is dressed plainly, with little makeup. She peers at the others through large glasses that seem to cover half her face. I was surprised she showed up. I knew this group session might be difficult for her but that it also might provide some sorely needed support.

"Well, I've never been married," she begins softly, "but I've had a number of, I guess you'd call them relationships. I've been hurt a lot. And maybe I've hurt others. My problem is. . . ." She stops suddenly for a moment and looks straight at me, as if for help. I gaze back but say nothing. Ginnie has to tell her own story.

"The reason I'm here is that I get physical with men fast. Too fast. And then it's no good anymore. They don't want me or I don't want them. I don't really know how to turn sex into love. It feels so great for a moment. I mean, you're in bed and it feels like it's forever. But it never is."

Ginnie is suddenly very self-conscious. She folds her arms across her chest and looks down. "I'm sorry. I shouldn't have said that."

There are several whispers of "No!" from the group, and I voice their support. "No, Ginnie, I'm glad you mentioned that. I think a number of people here can identify with those feelings." I am pleased that she opened up as much as she did. From our counseling sessions, I am aware of Ginnie's ongoing struggle. She wants to be a good girl and would like to live a chaste life, but she never has been able to maintain that for more than a few months at a time. Then it's out to the bars again for a series of one-night stands. Whenever a relationship seems to be taking hold, she does something to sabotage it. I suspect that the idea of a lasting relationship actually scares her to death, even though it inhabits her dreams.

I also know from our private sessions that Ginnie was sexually abused by her father. The only times she received his attention were when he came to her bedroom at night. This is how she learned to relate to men.

Realizing the depth of Ginnie's troubles, I know we won't solve them all tonight. I let her off the hook, moving on to Bonnie, a conservatively dressed woman of about forty. Bonnie is the last one in the circle.

"I've been divorced for about two years," Bonnie says. "It was a horrible marriage. I was verbally and emotionally abused for years. And I didn't realize it at the time. I just took it. It makes me mad now when I think about it."

"So what made you get the divorce?" asks Laurie.

"I found out he was having an affair—with another man. That was the last straw. It was a total shock, and I just couldn't deal with it. We separated almost immediately, and the divorce was fairly easy. But you know, it was the strangest thing. Once the divorce was final, I cried for three days. I was finally free from this . . . this monster, and I was grieving like it was the end of the world."

Bonnie goes on to talk about the relationships that came later. She felt a void in her life. In a way, she needed someone to take her husband's place. And she found one. She describes a current relationship with a man who also treats her poorly. He takes her for granted, always calls her at the last minute, and never takes her anywhere that costs him more than a few dollars, even though he has plenty of money. He continually promises her an increased commitment and eventual marriage, and yet he acts more and more distant. When Bonnie confronts him on some of these issue, he claims she is nagging and tells her to "get off his case."

"For about six months now," she says, "I've been trying to break up with him. And every time I do, every time I think it's finally over, he calls me and sweet-talks me into giving it another try. I'm so torn. I get angry and I say, 'We can't go on like this!' But deep inside, I need him. I miss him if we're not together. I can't stand not being with him."

"Can't live with him, can't live without him," says Margie. "I know the feeling." The others nod their assent.

Common Ground

As you can see, there are some major similarities in these people's stories. That's why I called the group together. It is common for people to isolate themselves in situations like these. Each feels that he or she possesses some major personality flaw and each feels alone. You noticed their comments, as I did: "I am so dumb!" "Why do I keep doing this?" "I know it's wrong, but . . . ."

Millions of people make the same mistakes. That doesn't mean it's not a problem. It does mean that the person is not abnormal. And it can be extremely therapeutic to get together with others and compare notes.

Let's take a look at the similarities of the people in our circle:

1. They are intensely drawn to a person or a particular kind of relationship, even to the point of irrationality. They seem almost out of control, much like those suffering from drug or alcohol addiction. Their "drug" involves relationships.
2. They seem unable to break the unhealthy cycle of relating. They tried to break up but couldn't. They divorced one jerk and began dating another. They repeated the same patterns, even though they knew just how badly those patterns end.
3. They seek personal fulfillment in a particular person or relationship. Each one in the group showed a lack of self-esteem, some more than others. They all were reaching out for some "missing piece" that would make them whole again.

This, I believe, is the major addiction of our era. The sexual revolution, the divorce epidemic, the technological isolation of individuals—all have contributed to a situation in which we long for healthy relationships and have no idea how to get them. The relationships we have are often twisted and unbalanced, beset by absurdly high expectations or low self-image. We are more aware than ever of our need for someone else, but too often we build up that need to messianic proportions.

Few are immune to addictive relationships—single and married, male and female, old and young, atheist and born-again Christian. You can be addicted to a husband or wife, boyfriend or girlfriend, parent, child, close friend, or someone you hardly know. The addiction can be fairly benign or obsessive and dangerous. In any case, we need to recognize relationship addiction as addiction, and treat it accordingly.

Movies such as *Fatal Attraction* depict the dark side of obsessive relationships, and we mourn over real-life stalker tragedies, but popular culture often describes even good relationships in addictive terms. We talk about being "crazy" about someone, implying that there's something wonderfully irrational about our attraction. If I "Can't Smile Without You," that is supposed to be a testimony of true love, not of dangerous attachment. When the artist then known as Prince barked "I Would Die 4 U," few of us thought about the problems of exalting a relationship to impossible levels. Even the most requested wedding song these days, Celine Dion's "Because You Loved Me," attributes the singer's entire well-being to the support of her lover. That's what love is supposed to be about, right?

Don't get me wrong. Love is great. And I'm not proposing some sort of coldly rational matchmaking system. But music, movies, books, and TV shows often tell us, "You are nothing if you aren't in love with someone. You have to be totally agog about this person, defying everything that makes sense just to be with this person." That kind of thinking plays well on the screen, but in real life it can lead to warped relationships.

Human love is a powerful thing. Ultimately it is a matter of two people giving their lives to each other, two people becoming one unit. But it needs to be balanced — both need to give — and healthy. When it's healthy, love builds up the lovers; it does not consume them.

Let's take a second look at the nature of addictive relationships before we tackle some of the variations on the theme.

Intense Attraction, to the Point of Irrationality

This kind of love hurts. It consumes a person. We talk of being "lovesick," longing for a person. In David's case, it's a temporary thing. He longs for a particular image of a woman he likes, but the reality never matches up. And Margie continues to crave a solid relationship with her "ladies' man" boyfriend, though she realizes he will probably never come through.

In cases of such intense attraction, we feel we must hang onto the person or keep pursuing the prize in spite of the pain involved. To maintain these unpromising or unhealthy relationships, we begin to sacrifice other relationships or to neglect aspects of our own lives. The objects of our affection begin to gain control over our lives. We become dependent on the brief highs in the relationship, even though it becomes harder and harder to obtain or maintain these highs.

Also, the objects of our affection sometimes realize the effect they have on us, and they milk it for all it's worth. Notice how several women in our circle bemoan the attitudes of the men they cling to. As David put it once in a session with me, "Men may be jerks, but women are stupid—stupid for letting men be jerks." David acknowledges that it can work the other way, too. More than once, a woman has played around with his heart precisely because he let her.

Strong love can be wonderful. But it can be dangerous—especially when it is not returned. Such intense attraction quickly throws a relationship out of balance. And a host of other difficulties follows.

Inability to Break the Unhealthy Cycle of Relating

The cocaine addict can reach a point when he hates what he's doing. The highs aren't high enough, his habit is expensive and dangerous, and it's ruining his life. But he's hooked. He can't get out, even though he recognizes how unhealthy it is. With drug, alcohol, and some other addictions, there's a physical element. Body chemistry changes, and withdrawal brings a bunch of physical symptoms. Relationship addiction does not have the same chemical hook, but the emotional hooks are powerful indeed. Virtually all of our circle members want to get out of unhealthy relationships or to change their patterns of relating—they just can't do it on their own. That's why they've come for counseling. They have sacrificed principles, convictions, friends, and self-respect to keep the unhealthy beast alive.

What amazes others as well as ourselves is that even when we are quite aware of how wrong a relationship is, we seem unable or unwilling to give it up. We gripe to our friends but ignore their advice. We tolerate treatment we swore we would never put up with, and we become miserable. Even if we seek professional help, we often discard the advice that we just spent our hard-earned dollars to hear. Addictive relationships are rooted in deep needs and can require deep therapy.

Devoted relationships are great. It's good to be loyal. But there's a major problem when you recognize that a relationship is unhealthy and a substantial part of you wants to get out of it, but you just can't.

Seeking Personal Fulfillment in a Particular Person or Relationship

What makes us act so irrationally? The fear of being alone is greater than the pain of the relationship. "A bad relationship is better than no relationship at all," we figure. (Isn't that essentially what Margie just said?) This implies that, by myself, I am unfulfilled, unworthy, and incapable of being happy.

Many people feel that there's something missing in their lives. And, as we've seen, popular culture has romanticized that— "You're Nobody Till Somebody Loves You." Romance takes on almost religious proportions. We are supposed to find the meaning of life in sex or romantic love.

Once again, don't get me wrong. Romantic love is a beautiful, mysterious thing, but too many people are searching for ultimate meaning in finite relationships. Their whole identity, their reason for living, is tied up in the affections or approval of another human being.

Interestingly, some scholars have defined idolatry as a root problem of addiction. The addict puts his "fix" (whatever that may be) in the place of God—worships it, serves it, depends on it, defines himself by it. As Gerald G. May writes in *Addiction and Grace*, "Spiritually, addiction is a deep-seated form of idolatry. The objects of our addictions become our false gods. These are what we worship, what we attend to, where we give our time and energy, instead of love."[1]

To some extent, human love does fulfill us. It can make us better people. But we can place absurd expectations on human relationships, and that's dangerous. You don't really "find yourself" in a relationship. You find yourself in yourself—perhaps in the context of a relationship. Don't go looking for your own soul in someone else's eyes.

CHAPTER TWO

Types of Addictive Relationships

ॐ

The lights are on
But you're not home
Your will is not your own
Your heart sweats
Your teeth grind
Another kiss and you'll be mine
You might as well admit it, you're addicted to love.[1]

IT'S NO SURPRISE THAT OUR SEX-CRAZY CULTURE CELEBRATES THIS KIND OF love addiction in song. Oh, to be free of any moral restraint. To indulge all passion. To escape into a never-never land without responsibility. And of course it's the ultimate fantasy to be with a sex partner who's "not home," has no will, and exists only for your pleasure—isn't it? It makes sense that the singer who popularized "Addicted to Love" appeared on the video with a cadre of women dressed exactly alike—tight dresses, slicked-back hair, high heels. They're human sex dolls, with no individuality, no personality, no will.

That's addiction for you. For the addict in the thrall of an addiction, all of life boils down to one thing—the fix. Whether that's cocaine, whiskey, or a date on Saturday night, that fix becomes the focus of life. Nothing else matters. No one else matters. The addict depersonalizes everyone, including himself or herself. The addict becomes a fix-seeking machine.

Can an addiction to a relationship—to a person—actually be depersonalizing? Yes. The relationship addict replaces the real person with an image, a false ideal of the person he or she adores. Addiction skews your vision of reality. Ironically, these false images make the wholeness the addict so desperately seeks impossible.

There are three major types of relationship addiction. They may look the same and share many symptoms, but the objects of desire are actually quite different.

"Love" Addiction

Some people are "in love with being in love." They find themselves in a series of budding romances that somehow fail to pan out. The actual relationship is usually too difficult to maintain once the euphoria of the romantic discovery has worn off. In some cases, the love addict demeans himself or herself in an effort to revive the fading feeling. A wife may allow her husband to have affairs, ignore her, insult her, even abuse her—all in the hope that he will someday love her again.

Dawn could be considered a love addict. The first one to speak up in the group, she had been divorced five years earlier and had experienced a series of painful relationships since then.

In private counseling, she told me that since the ninth grade she had never "been without someone." She was driven by the belief that someone out there would fulfill her and love her perfectly. Her marriage was promising at first, but it became deeply disappointing. Now she has found exciting love in an affair with a married man—but in the back of her mind she knows that this will end in disappointment and pain, too.

David, the lone male in the group, also seems addicted to the pursuit of a perfect love. While this type of addiction is much more prevalent in women, it also exists among men.

Like Dawn, David is looking for fulfillment in a romantic relationship. A million movies, TV shows, and dimestore novels promote the idea that romance brings fulfillment. As with most dangerous ideas, this is partly true. We can go back to Adam and Eve in the Bible and find the "missing rib" idea even there— we're lacking something until we find that missing piece. Many wedding ceremonies still incorporate this ancient notion that "the two become one flesh," which seems to imply that, individually, each person is worth only one-half.[2]

That's where the problem exists. There's nothing wrong with seeking a loving relationship where a certain fulfillment is found. But it gets dangerous when you depend on that relationship to make you a full person. A good loving relationship is the merger of two *whole* people. One plus one equals one. Let's not deal with fractions.

Addictions of this kind are usually built on a too-low opinion of self and a too-high opinion of the other person. Dawn, of course, had a low view of herself. She was willing to put up with all sorts of mistreatment because she figured she didn't deserve anything better. She drew her personal value from the men in her life—even when they beat her up.

But David shows us the other side. His self-image is fairly healthy, but he has built an idol called The Perfect Woman. Fueled by magazine layouts and rock videos, his mind has generated an image of the woman who will fulfill his life. He pursues women who have some of the desired traits, but he is disappointed when they don't measure up to his idol.

While he is in pursuit mode, David acts much the same way Dawn does. He doesn't have to deal with physical abuse, but he admits he's been used by several women he was devoted to at the time—stood up, taken advantage of, insulted. He allowed this to happen because he hadn't yet determined that she was not The One, so he could endure anything to keep her. Ironically, once he did win her affection, he realized her shortcomings and eased out of the relationship.

Sex Addiction

Sex addiction is either personal or impersonal. A common impersonal sex addition is pornography in various forms. It focuses on the individual's sexual pleasure, usually through masturbation.

Although it does involve other people—models, actors, prostitutes—it generally does not involve an ongoing relationship with these people. For that reason it lies beyond the scope of this book. (I would, however, recommend the excellent work by Patrick Carnes, *Out of the Shadows*.) (It must be mentioned that pornography addiction has devastating effects on the marriages and families of the addicts, as well. As much as the user of pornography seeks to isolate his compulsion, it spills over to the rest of his life and fouls his relationships.)

For many others, men and women alike, sex addiction is played out in personal relationships. They use other people for their own sexual compulsions.

Sex addiction is, on the surface, a quest for pleasure. But it can also be a quest for power or a method of self-sabotage. As with other drugs, the desire for sex draws people deeper and deeper in their quest for a greater and greater high. The addict finds that impersonal pornography doesn't please him anymore, so he indulges in new (sometimes dangerous or illegal) activities to attain his desired level of exhilaration and sexual release.

Often the pleasure is mingled with a sense of power. A man "conquers" a woman when he gets her into bed. A woman "controls" a man by tempting him into sexual relations. For some, this is the only power they have or the only power they consider important. It is not uncommon for late bloomers to blossom into promiscuity. Their self-image was stamped in junior high or high school as "ugly duckling," "nerd," or "undesirable." They may spend the rest of their lives trying to prove how wrong those labels were. How? By flaunting their newfound desirability, by seducing every person they can. Each new seduction is a triumph over the naysayers of their youth.

I know one young man who is successful and well-respected in his business and community. You would think he'd be very happy with where he is and where he's going. But there are two areas of his life in which he thinks he failed during high school. Though he was valedictorian and a popular student, he regrets that he never succeeded at sports or with girls. Today he's in his thirties and plays softball, volleyball, tennis, and basketball with a vengeance, often risking injury to prove he can excel. And, still single, he keeps dating the prettiest (and youngest) women he can, even if they're all wrong for him. He hasn't told me about the sexual aspects of his dating life, but his profile fits that of a certain type of sex addict. For them, it's not the sex act itself they crave, but a meaning attached to it. Sex is a victory, a vote of confidence, an emblem of power.

For Ginnie, sex equals love. The closest thing to love she experienced as a child was incestuous. And so she continues to attach love to sex. She exhibits all the symptoms of love addiction, except she seeks her fix through sex. And, from her story, it appears that she is terrified by the thought that love could be anything more than sex. Whenever a sexual relationship threatens to become more than that—if it moves in the direction of love—she kills it. Though she yearns to be loved, true love is uncharted terrain for her, and it scares her to death.

For others, and possibly for Ginnie, too, sex is a form of self-sabotage. They have deep feelings of self-hate and consider themselves unworthy of love. These feelings often come from childhood abuse. They think sex is dirty, and so sexual promiscuity is a way of playing in the mud. They often find an odd sense of justice in their behavior—they are punishing themselves for being bad by being bad. They know sex without love is demeaning and painful, but they feel they deserve the pain.

I recently saw a TV report on a young woman who suffered from something like this. The daughter of a famous actor, she became a stripper and then an actress in a pornographic film. She knew her behavior hurt her parents and her husband and even herself, but she seemed to be driven to continue it. Her reported conversations indicate that she thought very poorly of herself but delighted in the shame she brought to her famous father through her behavior. Ultimately she committed suicide, giving herself a death sentence for her sins.

That's an extreme case, to be sure. Most people who suffer from sex addiction are not nearly as public about it. In fact, many manage to keep it private until it grows out of control. They lead double lives, indulging their addiction and carrying on seemingly normal lives.

I once counseled a man named Frank. He was arrested for breaking into a woman's home at night and stealing her underwear. Because it was his first arrest, he was let off fairly easily. While the police called him a "weirdo" and several other choice names, the judge knew Frank needed not only punishment, but also some serious counseling.

To all appearances, Frank was no weirdo. He had a good job, a wife, and two children. Considered a moral person, he was even a Sunday school teacher in his church. But Frank had another life—a secret life no one else knew about. Frank grew up in an alcoholic home and swore he would never drink. But his inherited addictive tendencies came out in other ways. As a teenager, it was compulsive masturbation. As a young man, he sought a greater high and turned to pornography. He felt guilty each time he acted out and prayed that God would take away his lustful thoughts.

During this time, he had a steady girlfriend, but he never touched her sexually for fear of what he might do. He never discussed his problem with her, afraid she would reject him and his sinful ways.

Eventually Frank reasoned that his struggle stemmed from sexual frustration. Friends told him that he just needed to "score" and he'd feel better. But he clung to his convictions, believing that he shouldn't mistreat his girlfriend in that way. But what if they were married? Then sex would be all right and his problems would be solved—or so he figured.

At first it worked. For the first several months the marriage was a solution, but he couldn't help but notice that his sex drive was far stronger than his wife's. Still, this was far better than living with the guilt of the pornography and excessive masturbation.

Soon Frank began to masturbate again. This was a shock and disappointment to him because he assumed that all his sexual needs would be met by his wife. Yet he felt that he pushed her enough already to have sex a couple of times a week and didn't feel comfortable pushing her any more. So he decided to go back to his old pattern of using pornography and masturbating. This time he felt less guilt. *At least I'm not having an affair or hurting anyone,* he thought. But soon the pornography grew mundane, and masturbation seemed humiliating. He needed something more, he thought, a real woman. Once again, his strong convictions would not allow him to act on these thoughts. Instead, he fantasized about certain women he knew, seeking some connection with them.

One woman in particular became an obsession. He eventually followed her home and began a sexual ritual of returning after dark in order to watch her through her window while he imagined having sex with her.

Frank moved on to other women, then strangers, each time getting closer and closer without them ever knowing he was there. He began to call them and make obscene comments, climb trees to get closer looks, and eventually enter their homes while they were away. With each new phase the excitement grew, but his desire for greater connection also grew. Each risk he took heightened his fulfillment, but eventually led to greater risks.

Frank's behavior was becoming more and more self-destructive. The breaking-and-entering charge put an end to this cycle, at least for a time. When Frank saw how terrified the woman was to find him in her home, he was gripped with guilt. Somehow he had fantasized that their attraction was mutual.

Fortunately, Frank was caught. What would he have progressed to next? How far would his addiction have taken him? We don't know the answers to these questions in Frank's case, but newspapers are filled with the stories of other sex addicts. We can see how far their addictions have led.

Families have been torn apart, careers ruined, minds twisted.

But perhaps the greatest—and most common—destruction that sex addiction causes is the destruction of sexual satisfaction. Lost in a world of pornography, Frank could not be happy with his wife. She did not measure up to his fantasies. What should have been a beautiful thing—the expression of marital love through sexual intimacy—was poisoned. Unfortunately this has occurred in countless families.

A key word here is *attachment*. An addict attaches certain desirable qualities to a particular relationship or activity. These things then become fused together in the addict's mind. As we've seen, some people attach love to sex. So not only do they mistakenly feel loved when they're having sex, but they tend to feel unloved when they're not having sex. For some, it's power or control or self-worth that gets fused to their sexual behavior. The only time they can feel powerful, in control, or worth something is when they're having sex in some way. In Frank's case, as with many sex addicts, excitement was attached to pornography and voyeurism, and that removed the excitement from the rest of his life.

Addiction to a Person

Personal addiction is a matter of attaching one's wellbeing to a specific person. It is not "being in love with love" or being driven by sexual desire, though it may exhibit some of the same symptoms. In the other relationship addictions we've considered, the addict reduces all of life to a status, an emotion, or an activity. With personal addiction, it's all wrapped up in that special person. "If I don't see Bob today, I'll die."

When Bob is away, she feels desperately alone and out of control. When the object of her devotion is present, the world revolves around him. "It doesn't matter what I think, what I feel, what I want. I just want to make Bob happy." This is emotional dependency, and it can be dangerous.

Once again, our popular ideas of romance feed this dependency. When I was a kid, the Stylistics were singing "You are everything, and everything is you." That was no Hindu hymn; it was a love song. We regularly express our love in such lofty terms.

But if you're everything, then what am I? Where do I fit into the picture? The person addict says, "I don't." He or she loses a sense of self, while giving total devotion to the other. Needless to say, this makes for an unbalanced relationship. In the worst cases, the addicted partners endure terrible abuse yet keep coming back for more. They have no self-dignity to preserve. They cannot imagine living without their lovers/tormentors. They are convinced that they could never be loved by anyone else—nor would they want to be.

Joy is a perfect example of addiction to a person. As she explained to the circle, she was hanging onto a husband who wanted a divorce. She'd been with him since childhood and, while she acknowledged that the healthier thing might be to let him go and to start over, she did not know how to live without him.

I hesitate to do psychoanalysis based on news reports, but I suspect that O.J. Simpson had a person addiction to his ex-wife Nicole. The possessive attitude he reportedly displayed in his words and actions during their marriage seemed to continue in some form even after their breakup. Was O.J. addicted to Nicole? I can't say. But I have seen similar cases where person addiction became possessive and even violent.

Marriage isn't the only place we find person addiction. Dating relationships also can develop in that direction, as we saw with both Margie and Laurie. Margie has found the perfect man—or so she thinks. The trouble is that some other women have found him, too. He's a "ladies' man," with no immediate desire to settle down, and so the relationship is lopsided. Margie is crazy about him, ready to mortgage heart and soul for his exclusive affections. But obviously he's not that far along in his affection for her.

She fears (probably correctly) that if she presses the issue, she'll chase him away. So she stews in her addiction, happy for the few moments she can get, and miserable the rest of the time. Apparently he knows the rules of this game: he holds all the cards; she'll be there for him when he's ready.

In Laurie's case, the "rules" are even more one-sided. Laurie is addicted to her boss, who is "really sexy" even if he is "a real jerk." He has learned that he can use her addiction to get what he wants. He can mistreat her and she'll endure it; she just can't say no to him.

In all these cases we see how a person addiction devalues the addict while overvaluing the object of the addiction. "He's not worth it!" friends will say. "You deserve better!" But the addict's vision is warped; he or she can't see that.

And it's not just the addict who's hurt. The object of the addiction can get a bit warped, too. Laurie's boss is confirmed in his desire for a "winner take all" relationship. He knows nothing of the joy of give and take.

That's what addiction does. It tilts the playing field so all participants are at a disadvantage.

Person addiction also occurs in non-romantic relationships. Same-sex friendships (especially among women) can foster emotional dependencies. In these cases, a person's entire life—emotional state, self-confidence, energy—can hinge on a friend's presence or support.

Families also see their share of person addiction. Parents often get hooked on a child. They live their lives through their offspring and refuse to let go. Consider the stage mother who pushes a daughter into performing or the father who pressures his son to excel at sports. Often it seems as if the parents are fulfilling their own dreams of stardom and identifying too much with their children. But this can happen in many subtler ways as well. A parent may become overly involved emotionally with a child's teenage love life or job choices. Obviously a certain amount of concern and guidance is necessary, but it can cross the line of rationality. A child realizes, "This isn't about me or my choices anymore, is it? It's about you and what you wish you had done."

Person addiction isn't restricted to parents. A child can idolize an older sibling or a parent. I know several adults who are essentially controlled by their parents' opinions. They're convinced they could never make a good choice alone and desperately need the guidance of a perfect Mom or a do-no-wrong Dad. This too is a form of person addiction.

The Lure of Cybersex

A new variation on these themes has emerged, thanks to the rapidly growing Internet. Increasingly people feed their addiction to sex or love with their computers. Many spend hours in chat rooms hosted by online services, and others surf the Web for pornography.

Don was addicted to pornographic films and magazines as a young man but managed to kick the habit when he got married. But when he got a computer and went online, he checked out some of the sex sites he'd read about. His obsession rapidly returned.

He stayed up late, cruising site after site. His wife didn't suspect a thing. As far as she knew, he was working hard, doing research or maybe chatting with some computer pen pals. The problem was growing out of control and Don feared it would ruin his marriage—and his life.

That's when he came to me for counseling. "I managed to stop my pornography habit," he told me. "I thought I was through with that. But the stuff is so easy to find on the Net, I fell right back in. I'm hooked again."

Computer sex addiction appears to be a mixture of several other addictions. First of all, the computer itself can become an obsession. It is a gateway to worlds unknown. Microsoft was brilliant in developing its Windows commercials: "Where do you want to go today?" Download pictures from Mars, check stock prices in Tokyo, or visit a brothel in Amsterdam—it's all at your fingertips.

Computer addiction is becoming a major problem in our society. Its symptoms, as defined by the National Counseling Intervention Service, include users who:[3]

- Can't control time spent
- Suffer negative consequences from time spent
- Have an overdeveloped sense of the importance of the personal computer in their lives
- Use the computer as an outlet when depressed or sad

Now take your basic computer addiction and stir in the love addiction or sex addiction we've already described. The mixture is especially dangerous. Two types of problems emerge:

Love addiction that feeds off the fantasy of the chat rooms. On the Net, you can be whoever you want to be. This is especially enticing to people who are unsatisfied with who they are. In the chat room, a plain Jane can be a sultry Delilah. The 98-pound weakling can be Schwarzeneggar's twin. To the simple act of logging on, these love addicts attach power, fantasy, adventure, identity, and love. After experiencing all that on your computer screen, it's kind of hard to get back to the real world.

And that's exactly the problem. There's nothing wrong with chat rooms in and of themselves. People make friends, broaden their horizons, and learn new things through the Internet. But does your computer help you deal with real life or does it draw you away from it? If the Net becomes a fantasy world that demands more and more of your time, it's unhealthy for you.

Occasionally you'll read about a romance that started on the computer. After exchanging e-mail or rendezvousing in chat rooms, a couple finally meets and marries. (The same sort of thing has been happening among letter-writers for centuries.) In some cases, this pattern can overcome the focus on outward appearance that's so prevalent in society. People get to know each other's thoughts and feelings before judging appearance. That can lead to a deeper relationship than one just based on looks. But the Internet can also be used for deception. When this occurs, people get caught up in phony relationships. They may think they're developing a serious romance with a perfect partner, when in reality the partner they imagine doesn't really exist.

Sex addiction on-line feeds on pornography. The ease of access makes computer porn even more insidious than other forms. If a man wants to rent a video or buy a magazine, there's always the danger that someone will see him, which might ruin his reputation. For some people, that's enough to keep them honest. But the computer can pipe the images right into a home. *No one has to know.*

Cybersex addiction shares the characteristics of pornography addiction, but it's raised to a whole new level. The experience is becoming increasingly interactive—a user can order the kind of images he wants, and they're provided instantaneously. Essentially, the viewer becomes the director of his own pornographic film, which gives a strong illusion of power (which can add to the addictive pull).

Ironically, some are touting Internet porn as the ultimate "safe sex." Well, sure, if you're talking about viruses. But pornography addiction is anything but safe for those in its grip. The computer gives this addiction a powerful new weapon.

When he came for counseling, Don was looking for a program, some defined steps that would help him kick his new obsession. I gave him just one step: "Tell your wife."

Privacy is the incubator of sex addiction, and accountability is the best guard against it. Computer use is a very solitary activity—one person at a keyboard—and so it's easy to feed an addiction in private. (It's sad that the lure of sexual connections on the Net actually makes the user more and more alone.)

By contrast, accountability reconnects the cybersex addict to the real world. It's a major component of all twelve-step programs, and many have found it's all they need to keep them on course. Don needed to confess to his wife and get her help to monitor his Internet use. Otherwise, it would be too easy to succumb again.

Don did tell his wife, and she was stunned at first, just as he feared. But then she worked with him to defeat the problem. They succeeded. For Don, as with a number of others, the power of a real relationship helped to disarm the imaginary relationships of the cybersex world.

A Mixed Bag

Many people show symptoms of different types of addictions. This is not unusual. Love addiction, sex addiction, and person addiction are all related, and sometimes hard to distinguish. Social scientists find that cured drug addicts often gravitate toward other addictions, such as alcohol, cigarettes, or gambling. So it is with relationship addictions. In our group, Bonnie seems to have begun with a person addiction to her ex-husband. When she finally accepted her divorce, she soon settled into love addiction, needing to be in a relationship but moving quickly from man to man. Now she has settled on one man again, and again shows signs of a new person addiction as she endures his abuse.

Transitions like this are common. As people change, their needs change and their relationships change. But when new relationships don't pan out, despair leads to the pursuit of a new love—one that would be different and somehow more fulfilling this time. If only they could find the right person.

And so the addictive cycle continues.

CHAPTER THREE

Case Study: Sally

୫ঌ

SALLY CAME TO MY OFFICE AS AN ADDICTIVE ROMANCE WAS WINDING down. Her man was pulling away from her. His calls were less frequent. Alone on weekends, she drank. Her life was falling apart.

When did the trouble start? You might trace it to her upbringing. Sally's mother seemed paranoid about leaving her alone with her father. Sally never hugged him or had a loving relationship with him.

Or you might trace it to her marriage. In a gleeful rebellion against her parents, she married a much older man. She was happy that someone older and more educated would take an interest in her. He became her father figure, controlling her life. During their twenty-three years of marriage, he subtly chipped away at her self-esteem. She had to rely on him for everything. When someone asked her a question, she'd look to him for the answer. And he hit her whenever he thought it necessary.

Leave him? How could she do that? She had children to raise. She had no education. By herself, she was worth nothing—or such was the notion he had drummed into her. She began to take pills to ease the pain.

Or the trouble may have begun when she got a part-time job. The kids were grown, and they needed the money. Then it became a full-time job. Then she started to earn her college degree, one course at a time. She was becoming her own person—and he didn't like it. The marriage used to be about meeting his needs. Now she had needs of her own, and he felt threatened.

This caused turmoil in the family. In a fierce attempt to regain control of his family, he "disowned" their teenage daughter for a trivial offense. After taking every pill in the medicine cabinet, the girl ended up in the intensive care unit. Her psychiatrist urged that the father leave home. He did. But there was more trouble ahead.

A Law unto Himself

On the day her husband walked out, Sally visited her friend Jerry, a lawyer. He refused to handle her divorce but recommended a female lawyer across the street. Sally walked across the street, filed the papers, returned to Jerry's office, and received a dinner invitation. The dinner lasted all evening. Sally had another powerful man in her life.

He was a bit older, obviously well educated, and out of her league. Divorced three times, he was his own man now, living the good life. He wined and dine women in style. Sally knew he dated other women, but she dreamed that he would finally settle down with her.

"It was a relationship very much like my marriage," she says now, looking back. "I had him up on a pedestal. He was a lawyer, I was still a mere person. Why would he be interested in me? He treated me really nice. I was impressed. We went sailing often on his boat, but we never got together with his friends. He was ashamed of me." She became controlled by his opinion of her. She bought clothes she thought he would approve of. She tried to act in a way he would like. She was not herself with him. She wasn't sure anymore who "herself" was.

From the first night, the relationship was physical. That met a deep need within Sally—her need for loving touch that she lacked as a child—but she felt used by Jerry. He dropped her off early, complaining that he didn't feel well, and then (she'd learn later) see another woman. Sally loved the time she spent with him, but resented all the time without him. He stopped calling as often, and she began drinking more and more.

That's when she came to see me. She described her desperation, the ache of being by herself, her drunken binges each weekend. For a few more months she continued in a painful cycle. She would determine to stop seeing him, to stop giving in to him sexually. But then he'd call and she'd lose her resolve. "I'd hear his voice," she says, "and I'd forget all the meanness. He would say one word and all I had decided would go out the window." Once again, she was in a man's power.

Then he was gone for good, and her withdrawal was severe. "I wasn't happy with myself without someone else there. I needed a relationship." She had no friends at the time. People she knew from her marriage mostly abandoned her, and she didn't make any new friends while she was with Jerry. A few coworkers knew her casually, but not well enough to help much. The drinking got even worse. She was suicidal. I was afraid for her.

The Salesman

Sally met Richard at work. He was a salesman who visited the store. They struck up a friendship. About six months after her relationship with Jerry ended, Richard asked Sally out. She jumped at the opportunity. He was, quite literally, a life-saver. He was caring and attentive. A few months later, she learned he was married.

Still, Richard bolstered her self-esteem. "He told me how good I was for him. I did everything right. I did everything better than his wife. I cooked better, I cleaned better, I kept my car cleaner than she did. I soaked it up. I treated my kids better than she treated hers. I cleaned my cat's litter box better than she did. Can you imagine? But he was married to her."

Sally's weekends were still lonely. She managed to rendezvous with Richard as he traveled his sales circuit, in towns up to one hundred miles away. At that distance they could dine out and spend the evening in a motel. Sally drove out to meet him once or twice a week, flushed with excitement over their tryst. She drove home the next morning feeling awful.

Once again, the relationship was heavily physical. Sally longed to be held, to be loved, and it felt good in Richard's arms. The good feelings lasted through the night. Reality hit when the alarm went off.

"I felt like scum," she says. For two years she followed this pattern. Her life was all about drugs and drinking and driving the turnpike. She knew the relationship had no future, but she couldn't say no to it.

"Yet as much pain as it was, the feeling I had for those several hours was almost worth it."

In some ways, Richard was good for Sally. He didn't use her as badly as previous men in her life had. He took an interest in her family, and willingly became a part of her life—even though he had to exclude Sally from his own family life. Sally's kids liked him; they did things together. But they never knew he was married.

Sally dreamed that someday she and Richard would be together for good. She knew that was unlikely, and he had made no promises, but she kept dreaming. "I believe he really cared for me," she says now. "But he had a fine life with his wife and children. He wasn't going to leave them." And so she played a mental game of ping-pong, bouncing between hope and despair.

Richard took a vacation with his wife, and when he returned, things were different. He eased out of Sally's life. That sent her into more bouts of drinking and prescription drugs. She had stopped seeing me by this point, but she knew she needed help.

She was absent from work more than she was present. Her kids would call in and say she was sick, when really she was smashed out of her mind.

Getting Help

"I got tired of being sick, tired of drinking. A friend at work had mentioned that there was an evening rehab program in the area. I figured I could go there and still carry on my normal life. When I asked my friend about it, she said, 'No, you need detox.'" Sally made arrangements to go to a local institution for three days to dry out. With a blood-alcohol level of .40, she could hardly see straight on the drive there. She stayed for five weeks. When medical problems arose, she was transferred to a hospital. "I'm lucky I'm alive," she says. "They told me in the detox unit that I almost died."

After leaving the hospital, she got involved with Alcoholics Anonymous. She attends AA meetings regularly and speaks highly of the program. It has contributed greatly to her healing.

As she sits here and tells her story, she has been clean and sober for one year, one month, and nine days. The drying-out process also has given her strength to confront her tendencies toward addictive relationships. She has a new self-esteem she never had before.

"Boy, do I like myself!" she says. "I don't have a romantic relationship with anybody right now, but I've made a lot of friends in the program. And I've learned I can do things on my own. I'm not afraid to be alone. It's really a neat feeling—I feel worthwhile. I'm not looking for a romance now. If it comes along, I'll consider it, but I'm not looking for it. I'm okay by myself."

Recently Sally had some legal business, and she had to see Jerry, her old lover/lawyer. She reports that she did so without a pang of regret. This man had held power over her—his voice could melt all her resolve. She had allowed him to use her in the past, but now there was no feeling for him. Not even anger. They went about their business and she left. No longing looks. No heartfelt sighs. Nothing.

What's the difference between then and now? "I'm much more sure of myself," she explains. "I have my self-esteem back. I'm important. I count." It's good to hear her say that.

Evaluation

What type of relationship addiction did Sally have? I'd say she had them all, with various substance addictions thrown in. She seems to have been a victim of love hunger since childhood. Her father's distance, her mother's paranoia, and her husband's abuse combined to create a very needy woman.

These needs came out physically in her sexual relations with the various men in her life. She complained that her husband would only touch her when he wanted to, that he cared little for her sexual needs. Although later affairs were more passionate, the same pattern seemed to be in place. She wanted love and offered sex. She was used and disappointed. This is a common pattern for female sex addicts.

Nevertheless, she longed for more than sex. It was only a steppingstone to a deeper relationship—or so she hoped. Her low self-esteem made her *need* to be with somebody. The affair with the lawyer was both exhilarating and defeating. His status lifted her up for a time, but then dashed her to the ground when she realized he would never marry her. She gave up all her personal boundaries with both Jerry and Richard. Even though Richard showed a genuine love for her, they still met on his terms, and she demeaned herself with those long, inebriated drives. "I'm nobody unless somebody loves me" quickly turned into "I'll do whatever I have to do to win and keep someone's love." That's the downward spiral of the love addict, seeking to *be* somebody by being *with* somebody.

Sally showed signs of person addiction as well. Her lengthy stay in an abusive marriage is the first example. She says her husband "chipped away" at her self-esteem, to the point where she no longer had opinions of her own. Her husband was her god. When she finally broke free from him, with a few early stabs at self-awareness, she quickly chose a new god to worship. Jerry was "out of her league," and she was tickled that somebody like that would pay attention to her. She willingly closed her eyes to his philandering and dreamed of an eventual paradise with him. Her relationship with Richard was just a fantasy. After all, that's what an extramarital affair is. There's none of the commitment and hard work required in a truly loving relationship. Still, Sally viewed him as a savior of sorts. He helped her when she needed it—and so she conveniently forgot the fact that he was an unfaithful husband. This willful ignorance of the flaws of one's lover is a hallmark of person addiction.

Sometimes a person has to hit bottom before healing can start. That seemed to be Sally's situation. Ironically, it was probably the crisis of her chemical dependency that forced her to look at the self-esteem issues that spawned her relationship addictions. That dependency also nearly killed her.

She went back to square one. She took a hard look at her basic assumptions about herself. And, for now, she's looking and sounding good. She knows relapse is possible. She knows there are dangerous times ahead. But she is arming herself with the awareness of her own needs and an appreciation of her own value.

CHAPTER FOUR

Characteristics of Addictive Relationships

⨯⧜

J UST WHEN ARE YOU ADDICTED? IS A WIFE WHO STAYS IN A DIFFICULT
marriage demonstrating sacrificial love or is she addicted to the
relationship?

What about a single woman who prefers to go out with a
man that she is not too thrilled about rather than staying home on
a Saturday night?

Or a man who has had twelve relationships in the past five
years? Is he an addict or just a man who likes to date?

And how about a woman who calls her mother every day,
sometimes two or three times a day, and tells her every detail
of her life—often before she tells her own husband? Is this
woman addicted to that maternal relationship or is she just a
good daughter?

These distinctions can be elusive without a look at the characteristics of addictive relationships. If we define addiction as that
drive to be with and stay with a particular person, then almost
every committed relationship has some element of addiction.
Likewise, when love is defined as the desire to commit and sacrifice your own good for the good of another, there is also some
element of true love associated with most addictive relationships.

So we seem to have a continuum between lovingly healthy relationships and severely addicted ones. Almost all romances and good friendships fall somewhere between the two. So what's the difference? Where is the danger point on that scale? Where do Romeo and Juliet turn into . . . well, Romeo and Juliet? That is, when does tender love become suicidal angst?

Characteristics of an Addictive Relationship

There may be no specific dividing line on that continuum between healthy and unhealthy relationships. But as we observe relationships on both ends of the spectrum, we see a number of basic differences between them. Then, as we get a picture of what healthy and unhealthy relationships look like, we can better evaluate the health of our relationships. You don't need to sound the alarm if you recognize only one or two of these symptoms in your own relationships, but if the overall pattern looks familiar . . . well, it's a good thing you're reading this book.

1. Free Choice vs. Compulsion
In a truly loving relationship, the partners freely choose to be with each other, to be associated with each other, to love each other. In an unhealthy addictive relationship, the free choice is replaced by compulsion. You simply *have* to be with that person, whether you really *want* to or not.[1]

Compare this situation to that of the cocaine addict. By controlling the user's mind and emotions, the drug inhibits the freedom to choose. In a way, the addict makes a free choice with every snort, but the drug itself biologically stacks the deck in favor of drug use. The more you choose the drug, the more it controls you, and the less freedom you actually enjoy.

So it is with the addictive relationship. The biology is slightly different, but the principle remains. Your brain gets used to certain impulses from the relationship. In a way, they drive a rut into the pathways of your mind. You may *think* you're making choices, but the more involved you get in the relationship, the more it controls your life. You feel powerless to break it off, and therefore your freedom of choice is limited. The deeper the relationship gets, the more control it has over your life.

In a healthy relationship, you are still drawn to the person and willing to sacrifice in order to make it work, but you maintain objectivity. Your judgment overrides your emotions, which helps you remain in control of your choices. This means that you hold the other person accountable for his or her actions. You won't stand for mistreatment, and you will recognize when your love isn't returned.

Becky and Bob dated for a while and grew close quickly. As their relationship developed, Becky noticed Bob taking her more and more for granted. He began to call at the last minute or just stop by and then hang around watching TV. He made himself at home with her, eating her food and taking advantage of her generous nature. He also made it clear that he expected a sexual relationship. When she complained that they never went out anymore, he usually commented on his need to save money, and he promised some special date on an unspecified later occasion. In spite of Bob's treatment, Becky found herself so emotionally drawn to him that she dared not risk making him mad. She continued to feed and wait on him whenever he came over. But Becky found that the more she gave, the more empty she felt inside—especially after giving in to him sexually. In order to numb this uneasy feeling, she tried harder and harder to show him how much she loved him, hoping that he would try harder to love her. But in reality, other than a few times when she saw glimmers of hope, the relationship only worsened.

With Becky feeling utterly frustrated about the relationship, and with friends now beginning to question what she saw in Bob, she determined to break it off. Yet whenever she rehearsed the breakup, she only convinced herself that "now is not a good time" or "if I wait a bit longer, perhaps he'll change." Over a period of months, instead of breaking off with Bob,

Becky actually grew even more emotionally dependent. She detached from many of her previous friends because she had less and less time for them, and because she tired of hearing their negative opinions about Bob.

The relationship finally ended about a year later when Bob began seeing someone else. Becky was devastated. Adding to her depression over the loss of this relationship was the fact that she had lost contact with almost all of her former friends. She felt emotionally and spiritually isolated.

Why did Becky stay with Bob so long? Was she in love with him? Was she objective about the relationship or was she driven by an empty feeling inside which limited her ability to choose to pursue (or not pursue) this relationship?

You may be thinking, *What Becky put up with was nothing in comparison to what I've gone through.* Indeed there are far more severe stories to tell. For many, the compulsion to stay in the relationship at any cost has led to the toleration of physical, sexual, and emotional abuse. As we sink deeper and deeper into the relationship, the power of the compulsive drive seems to deepen. We end up compromising most of our standards, beliefs, and values just to maintain the very thing in our life that is hurting us the most.

2. Mutual Support vs. Attempt to Rescue

Have you ever known people who always seemed to date beneath themselves? The sweet, innocent girl who dates the drug addict? The upstanding young man who goes out with the emotional wreck? Certainly we shouldn't overgeneralize these cases, and the whole concept of someone being "beneath" someone else is a dangerous one. But situations like this are often unhealthy because they are unbalanced from the start. The motivation underlying such relationships is often not love at all, but pity, pride, or a compulsive need to save someone.

In healthy relationships, both partners help each other function, grow, and "be all they can be." In addictive relationships, one person often tries to rescue, fix, reform, save, or at least enable the other. There is a constant tilt to the relationship. One is always in need; the other needs to be needed. They become dependent on each other in this lopsided state, which we call *codependency*.

I knew a woman in college who was a classic codependent. Though she was religious, she always gravitated toward guys with shady backgrounds. I found this especially frustrating because I was attracted to her myself, but she would never go out with me because I wasn't needy enough. She was into what I called "missionary relationships." I watched as she took a friend of mine under her wing. He was converted in prison, while serving time for armed robbery and drug possession. She was determined to help him in his spiritual development. But their spiritual intimacy quickly became physical, and soon they were romantically involved.

I don't know what happened to that relationship. Perhaps it lasted. Perhaps he grew in his faith with her help, and maybe they learned to treat each other as partners. But I doubt it.

You see, that's the problem with codependency. It is built on one's need and the other's need-meeting. What happens when the new convert grows into spiritual maturity? What does the "missionary" do then? The whole basis of the relationship has shifted. She isn't needed anymore, at least not in the same way.

Ray told me of his dating relationship with a woman who recently had been divorced. When he met her, she was still devastated by her husband's desertion. Ray was able to bring her some joy and to rebuild her confidence.

Though she was determined not to rush into a rebound relationship, she was emotionally needy, and Ray was ready to meet her needs. He thrived on this need-meeting. The friendship moved quickly into a romance. "It was important for her to feel desirable again," Ray figured. He loved the thought that he was restoring her to wholeness.

A funny thing happened. She became whole again. And then

she didn't need him anymore. The tilted ground on which their romance rested had become level, and that changed everything. Fortunately, they both realized this and broke up rather amicably. There's an interesting footnote to this story. Within a year after her breakup with Ray, the woman married a man who had suffered a painful divorce himself. She had found someone with whom she could engage in mutual support.

And Ray's next relationship? A struggling single mother.

Codependents need dependents. The examples here have been rather mild. We could find many cases of alcoholics or drug abusers and their codependent spouses. The codependent gets hooked on helping the dependent.

The problem is that the whole relationship is built on crisis. The rescuer is in a Catch-22 situation. If he or she succeeds in rescuing the dependent, restoring the needy person to health, that will shake the relationship. If the once-dependent partner doesn't need any more help, the rescuer can't get high on helping any more. So, subconsciously, the rescuer has a vested interest in keeping the dependent. The codependent enters into the addictive cycle.

3. Objectivity vs. Rose-colored Glasses

In a healthy relationship, both partners recognize the value and shortcomings of the other. In an addictive relationship, one partner denies any negative aspects of the other. "He's perfect," a woman might say, "the man of my dreams." Her friend may see a million things wrong with him, but the woman in love is blind to all that.

"Love is blind." So goes the old adage. But if attraction is going to grow into anything healthy over the long term, it had better open its eyes.

I'm not trashing the idea of maintaining a "positive mental attitude." It is good to look for the positive aspects of the people we meet. But we have to be objective. It's naive and dangerous to ignore the negative.

Such rose-colored glasses are common when people are infatuated. You may know this feeling. "You're wonderful. You're the answer to all my problems. You're exactly what I've been looking for all my life." This is a natural phase that usually occurs at the start of a relationship.

M. Scott Peck describes the "myth of romantic love" in this way: "We have met the person for whom all the heavens intended us and, since the match is perfect, we will then be able to satisfy all of each other's needs forever and ever."[2]

We willingly put aside the problems that arise. We're in love. "I only have eyes for you." As I said, this is a natural feeling that occurs in many lives. For a time, it's healthy and fun. In fact, without such temporary blindness, men and women might never get together. Peck wryly adds that the myth of romantic love, while it's a "dreadful lie" may be "a necessary lie, in that it ensures the survival of the species by its encouragement and seeming validation of the falling-in-love experience that traps us into marriage."[3]

The problem occurs when infatuation refuses to grow up. While "falling in love" is a natural phase, so is the fading of those feelings. Healthy relationships grow into an objective, responsible love that weathers the storms of life. As love matures, the partners begin to see each other's bad side—and we *all* have one.

Scholars liken infatuation to the development stage of a two-year-old. You've heard of the "terrible twos." What makes that age so terrible is that the child usually feels omnipotent. The child is walking and talking and Mom and Dad are still responding to every need.

During that year, the child learns that there are limits. Mom and Dad are free agents, not always predictable—and that can be very disappointing. The child can't do everything he or she sets out to do. It's a sobering time, but one that's necessary for the child's growth. You may have seen children who get to be five or six and still act like they're in the terrible twos. They're spoiled rotten. They have never made that break from Mom and

Dad. They have never learned their limits. It's obvious that their development is stunted.

Similarly, the infatuated person feels omnipotent. He or she is walking on air. Let the world rush past. Maybe millions of people go by, but they all disappear from view, 'cause I only have eyes for you. You and me against the world. I got you, babe—and nothing else matters.

But growth means opening one's eyes to the rest of the world. Growth means re-establishing a certain distance from the other person. Growth means understanding the limits of that person and the borders of that relationship. If that growth does not occur, the relationship is stunted. It can remain in that infantile state for many years.

I counseled a couple who seemed to stay in this infatuation stage too long. Even after a year of dating, they seemed very much "in love." They couldn't keep their hands off each other. Every time I saw them, they were all googly-eyed, exchanging loving glances or nibbling an ear or pecking a cheek.

That's cute behavior. Puppy love. But it surprised me that they were still at this point after being together a year. I talked with them soon after they were engaged, and asked them about positive and negative characteristics of each other. The answers I got were all positive. "I couldn't live without her." "When he's away from me, I feel empty inside, and when he's near I'm complete."

Sounds wonderful, right? I'm glad my wife wasn't present. She might say, "Why don't you ever talk about me like that? Why don't you love me in that way?"

But that misses the point of what true love is. Love doesn't mean "I can't live without you; you're all I could ever dream of." Love means that I recognize your good points and bad points, and I entrust you with mine. I still commit myself to be true to you, to serve and be served, to honor and be honored.

Too many couples panic when the infatuation fades. "We're falling out of love!" But the fact is, that's when true love *begins* to grow. In unhealthy relationships, people reach for the rose-colored glasses. "If I allow myself to see how bad he is, that will destroy the feelings that make me feel so good." In healthy relationships, people risk honesty—both in sharing and seeing—in order to grow into a more mature love.

Mature love also means that the partners hold each other accountable for their actions. If your partner doesn't show up for an important date, what are you going to do? You could make excuses for your partner. You could accept your partner's flimsy excuses without a word of protest. That's the rose-colored glasses method.

But a healthy love would confront the situation in a firm but forgiving way. "That date was very important to me. It hurt me a lot that you didn't show up. But besides my own pain, I'm concerned about our relationship. It makes me think that you don't care about us. If your excuse is true, I forgive you, but you can't keep standing me up like that. That's not the kind of relationship that's good for either of us."

By stepping back and viewing things objectively, you can make wise decisions about what's good for you, your partner, and the relationship.

4. Exclusive Attention vs. Balance with Other Friends

"What happened to Ricki? She used to be so active in our singles group. She had many friends of both sexes who supported her and received support from her as we all went through the various crises of singleness. We cheered her on as she told us of a promising new relationship in her life. Tony was attentive, sensitive to her needs, showering her with flowers, taking her to places she loved. She had dated more than her share of skunks, and we were glad for her good fortune.

"Then we stopped seeing her. She begged out of our group activities. A few of us phoned her and were treated politely, but Ricki seemed distant. Sue managed to arrange a shopping trip with her, and she reported that Ricki was constantly worried about what Tony would think of this dress, that blouse, those stockings. The conversation revolved around Tony. Ricki, it seemed, had no other life.

"That was six years ago. We all lost touch with her."

Recently, Ricki called Sue. They got together over coffee at a local diner, and Ricki unfolded her story. She married Tony. His constant attention won her over; she felt loved, desired, prized. She was his trophy.

But Tony was the jealous type, and soon she became a prisoner in her own home. His jealousy made her sever ties with the singles group. Even while they were dating, he was suspicious of those friendships and pressured her to break them. Then, when they married, the jealousy got worse. He grilled her about any contact she had with anyone. She was even afraid to speak to the mailman.

She had a child and gained a great deal of weight. She felt undesirable, and Tony apparently thought so, too. Now the child was his prize, and Ricki was just a nurse. He went on long business trips and carried on affairs with little attempt to hide them, but he kept checking up on Ricki. He still discouraged any outside friendships.

There she was, locked in a bad marriage. She had cut herself off from the friends who could help her; she felt unworthy of new friendships; and she had a baby to take care of. She told Sue about how Tony, in a drunken rage, had pulled out a gun and threatened her. "If you ever fool around on me. . . ." That was when she knew she had to get out.

Sue gave her encouragement and some practical advice, but there was a wall between them. Ricki cut herself off from her closest friends, and it wasn't easy to restore those friendships. She moved out and divorced Tony, but never came back to the church or the singles group.

That's an extreme case, but its patterns are not unusual. You may know some people with similar stories. A jealous boyfriend or girlfriend. Severed friendships. An exclusive focus on that one relationship. Then, often, abuse of the relationship.

Exclusivity is not always so one-sided, not always the result of jealousy. Sometimes two people feel so passionately about each other that they both want to spend all their time together. Their other friendships slip away. Suddenly the guy you play basketball with on Thursday nights can't make it. He's out with his girlfriend. Suddenly the girl in the theater group has to drop out of the cast because she's spending all her time with her new boyfriend.

Like infatuation, this phase is natural. But when it goes on for too long, it gets dangerous. The implication behind exclusive relationships is this: Two people in love can meet all of each other's needs. But it isn't true! That guy needs to play basketball—and her jump shot is lousy. She needs to act, but he doesn't know Tennessee Williams from Mississippi mud pie. To be whole, those two people need to do the things they love, and they need to maintain the friendships that have supported them. Yes, there will be some adjustments as the couple grows closer. Each of their schedules will shift a bit as they make time to be together. But neither partner needs to have complete dibs on the other. That's unwholesome and unhealthy.

In a healthy relationship, both partners know that they have priority but not exclusivity in the other's life. Many needs are met within the relationship, but others are met outside it. Each partner can and should share friends with the other, but long-time friendships should not threaten a romantic relationship.

I have healthy and unhealthy examples from my own life. As I was recovering from my divorce, I began to date someone who met a lot of my needs. And I was needy. It was sort of a "tick on a dog" relationship. I latched on to her and began to take and take and take. She was a nurturing person, so she was very happy to give and give and give. (This was one of those rescue relationships that can be therapeutic for a time but seldom lasts.)

We began to see each other every day. She would cook dinner for me regularly, but sometimes I had to work until late at night. Even then, I'd get home and call her immediately. She would say, "Why don't you come over, even for a few minutes. I haven't seen you all day. I miss you. I'd like to be with you." Of course, I felt the same way.

So we began to spend all our time together, which quickly excluded other relationships. I didn't go fishing with the guys any more because I wanted to be with her (and she wasn't interested in fishing). My other activities and friendships were preempted because I was "in love" with this woman.

As you might guess, this relationship didn't last. As I grew back to emotional health, I didn't need her as much. And I became aware that our whole relationship was based on my need. We broke up, with considerable pain for both of us.

A few years later I began another relationship. By this time I had gained a number of new friends, I was involved heavily in my church, and I'd begun to work in Fresh Start, a divorce recovery program. I was very interested in this new woman, but she was busy, too. We could only see each other every two or three weeks.

As our relationship grew, we spent more and more time together, but neither of us scrapped our old friendships. We recognized that those friendships and activities were part of who we were and part of what we brought to each other. We each allowed the other to spend that necessary time with other friends.

That woman is now my wife. To this day, we maintain some separate friendships. We meet many of each other's needs, but there are other social and recreational needs we can't meet for each other. We don't have to.

5. Trust vs. Jealousy

"Where were you?"

"Who were you with?"

"I saw the way you looked at her! What's going on?"

"Why can't we be together more often? Is there someone else?"

Jealousy is an ugly monster. It can infest a relationship and destroy it. Jealousy is born of insecurity and desire. It is completely unreasonable. Wild charges are made, exposing deep feelings of pain or fear. If you've been jealous within a relationship, you know how it gnaws at you, defying your attempts to control it. If your partner has been the jealous one, you know how frustrating it can be to sidestep the traps that monster sets.

The jealous person fears that his or her partner will leave for someone more beautiful, more interesting, more suitable, or more financially stable. This possibility creates a panic and results in irrational attempts to control the partner's life. This can chase the partner away, unless the partner is addicted, too.

Underlying the jealousy is the convoluted logic of relationship addiction. "I'm not worth anything. By myself I'm miserable. But with this other person by my side, I'm worth something, I'm happy. I need this person. But since I'm not worth anything, my partner is bound to find someone else who is worth more. That person will steal my partner away, and that will make me miserable again. So I need to prepare for that, or guard against that, and keep my partner from finding anyone else." In the process, everyone becomes miserable. The jealous person fulfills his or her own prophecy, in a way. Convinced of their own unworthiness, jealous people sabotage whatever happiness is within their grasp.

I knew a woman who was overcome by jealousy about her boyfriend. Every day Ann would call Brian and ask about his day. (That's nice; nothing wrong so far.) "So, what did you do today?" she'd ask.

The broad question would usually bring a vague answer. "Oh, nothing much. I went to work, worked on some projects, went home." (Anything objectionable there? No, but Ann had to keep digging for something.)

"Did you talk to anybody today?"

"Sure," Brian would answer. "We had some meetings, and a bunch of us went to lunch." (A bunch of us? What is he hiding?)

"Oh," Ann would say gently. "Who all did you talk to?"

"At work? Or at lunch? No one special. Joe and Pete in my

office. And Mr. Williams stopped in about that project."
(Nothing yet.)

"Well, who was at lunch?"

"Oh, the guys. You know. Barry from the mailroom and Carl and Art and Sally." (Bingo!)

"Sally? Did you talk with her?"

"Yeah, a little."

"About what?"

Brian would pause as he tried to remember the trivial conversation of earlier that day—or, as she interpreted it, to come up with a good story. "I don't know. About the job mostly."

"What did you say about the job?"

By this time, Brian would be a bit peeved. "I don't know, Ann. It was a silly conversation over lunch, okay? I don't remember what we said. It wasn't important." (Right.)

"Well, you don't have to get upset. I'm just interested in your life. If you don't want me to be interested . . . ." (I must be onto something, Ann figures. He's getting defensive.)

"No, Ann, I'm glad you're interested in my life. I'm interested in yours, too."

"So, Brian, do you have lunch with Sally very often?"

"No! Well, yes, but no. It's not that. It's just a bunch of us. We work together. Sally's one of the group." (Brian has stepped into the quicksand.)

"But you talk with her. Do you like talking with Sally?"

"No!"

"So she forces herself on you."

"No, it's not like that! I talk to everyone. Sally happened to sit across from me." (Oops. A detail better left unsaid.)

"And do you think that was an accident?"

"What?"

"That Sally sat across from you. I'm a woman; I know these things. She's after you, Brian, and I don't like it. I don't think you ought to talk to Sally anymore."

"But Ann—"

"Promise me you won't talk to Sally."

"But I work with—"

"Who's more important to you, Sally or me?"

"You, of course, but—"

"Well, I'm not so sure about that. You seem to be standing up for her. Was she the one working late with you last Thursday when you were late to dinner?"

"There was a bunch of us."

"I've heard that before."

And suddenly all the old laundry gets taken out and spread across the relationship. Ann has turned a friendly chat into the Spanish Inquisition. She has decided that this working colleague is The Other Woman. She has assumed that a casual lunch with coworkers amounted to a private romantic tryst.

While I changed a few of the details, this conversation is typical of the ones Ann and Brian told me about in counseling. They would have huge fights over minor items like this, and then get back together, and the jealous rage would build again.

Obviously, this was not a healthy relationship. They had to learn to trust each other. Ann, especially, had to learn to trust Brian. But more than that, she had to trust that she herself was good enough for Brian. Her need to control Brian's life came out of a lack of appreciation for her own life.

The fact is, Brian could have been dating Sally. Ann's irrational suspicions may have been right. The problem was that the very thought threw Ann into a panic. How would she live without him? If she were convinced that she could live quite well without him, there would be no such panic. She could still express her love for Brian and her desire for a committed relationship, but she would not react with desperation to the possibility that he might choose otherwise. Her life would go on, regardless.

In some cases, the addicted person is the object of the partner's jealousy. This was the case with Ricki. She should have seen signs of a dangerous possessiveness in Tony, but she was blind to it. Her lack of self-appreciation made her crave the appreciation he was showing, even if that made her a trophy and dehumanized her.

One of the key points of Christianity is Jesus' command: "Love your neighbor as yourself." It gives us crucial insight into the reciprocal nature of relationships. The antidote for jealousy is to trust your partner as you trust yourself. Your partner may disappoint you, may hurt you, may run off with a coworker, but you need to trust yourself to be okay by yourself. That will help you avoid relationships with those who don't deserve trust (like Tony), and it will pave the way for open, trusting communication.

6. Recovery vs. Continuing Dysfunctions

People who get into addictive relationships often have come from dysfunctional family patterns. A dysfunction, quite simply, is when something doesn't work as it should. In fact, dysfunctions are usually patterns that go against the proper working of a person or a family. If I get a flat tire, that's a problem. I might even consider it a crisis. And we could probably call it a misfunction. The tire, being flat, isn't doing what a tire should. But I stop and fix it and drive on.

But if my car is badly out of alignment, that's another thing. It affects my steering, the car wobbles to the right as I drive, and my tires get worn quickly on one side, leading to more flat tires. This might be considered a dysfunction. It's not just one thing that goes wrong. The whole system goes out of whack.

So it is with families. Family crises can be dealt with and recovered from—in time. But dysfunctions last. The family system is supposed to work a certain way: love, nurture, discipline, education, and so on. These are the family's systems. If the parents are divorced, and the children see their father only once a month, that threatens to mess up the family system. If the parents are always fighting or if they never talk to each other, they are modeling unhealthy behaviors for their children. The family isn't working as it should. If one parent is an alcoholic, and the children are forced to go through the cycles of addiction, that will also create basic problems in the way the family works. Obviously, if there is spouse abuse or child abuse, sexual or otherwise, that will create long-term problems in the children's lives.

Unless a person makes a concerted effort to recover from those family dysfunctions, he or she is liable to repeat those errors in future relationships. Messed-up children often become messed-up adults and messed-up parents, continuing the cycle.

Dawn and Ginnie, from our circle, illustrate this point. Dawn grew up with an alcoholic father and fought all her life for his affection. She's still fighting for it, only now she seeks it from other men. She jumps at the promise of affection from the men she dates and tends to scare them away with her zeal.

Ginnie's case is even more severe. Sexually abused by her father, she learned to equate sex with love. That was the only attention her father ever gave her. So now she, too, seeks fatherly affection, but she seeks it through sex—and is consistently disappointed.

Healing *is* possible. People can recover from a dysfunctional past, but it takes some hard work and a lot of help. Dawn and Ginnie are like countless others who seek counseling to dig up their past and lay it to rest again. But it doesn't happen overnight.

In addictive relationships, people tend to come from dysfunctional backgrounds—and tend not to deal with them. They continue to deny their deep-seated need even as it affects every choice they make. In healthy relationships, people have dealt with their dysfunction or are diligently working through it.

7. Healthy Independence vs. Overdependence
People who get into addictive relationships tend to be emotionally dependent people. That is, they have a great inner drive to be connected with someone.

We all need other people; that's normal. But overdependent people feel they need people in their lives all the time. Or they want to have a special relationship with a particular person all the time. When they're by themselves, they feel lonely and empty. This creates a certain desperation to be with someone—anyone. And that leads to bad relationship choices. When they do find someone to hook up with, their desperation tends to overburden the relationship. They demand too much.

The people in our circle exhibited a lot of overdependence. "He's, like, inside of me. I need him," said Dawn. "I needed the guy more than he needed me," explained Margie. "I want to be with him all the time," Laurie added. This is the language of overdependence.

Each woman would be better off if she could learn to embrace a healthy independence. "I'm fine on my own. If you want me, come and get me. I'm going to the movies Saturday; if you'd like, you can join me." That attitude would revolutionize their relationships.

8. A Growing Relationship vs. a Love-hate Cycle

"He's a really sexy guy," says Laurie, "but he's a real jerk, too." That kind of good-news/bad-news joke is common to addictive relationships. You love him, you hate him, but you can't get away from him. You *need* him.

A friend in college went through that cycle regularly, and brought everyone else on that roller-coaster with her. Cristy would get mad at her boyfriend. For two days she would bad-mouth him to all her friends. "I don't know why I ever went out with him! He is so wrong for me! He has no compassion, no sensitivity! I don't care if I ever see him again!"

Then she'd see him again.

For the next few days, she'd be happier than ever. He was wonderful, perfect, the man of her dreams.

Until they had another fight. Then he became a nightmare again.

Some people seem to thrive on such volatile relationships. But the crucial question is: Where is the relationship going? Are the two people growing together with each new disagreement?

Or are they just replaying the same old issues? How does the couple handle conflict? Are they resolving it through a healthy give-and-take? Or are they at an impasse, with neither giving in? When they do get back together, is it because they've decided to make the necessary compromises to work out their problem? Or do they just "need" each other so much that they decide to ignore the problem until it flares up again?

Every relationship has its disagreements. But in a healthy relationship, the partners talk through the problems, work through them, learn through them, learn about each other, learn about themselves, and move on. That's growth. That may mean the relationship reaches a higher level of understanding and commitment. Or it may mean the partners decide the romantic relationship isn't worth pursuing. Either way, the individuals are growing as they deal with their conflicts.

Addictive relationships are characterized by unresolved conflicts. Any disagreement becomes a stumbling block. This goes along with the rose-colored glasses routine. You can't admit there might be a problem, so you sweep it under the rug. You keep sweeping it under the rug until one day it's so big you trip over it and fall flat on your face. The point is that conflicts need to be dealt with. Refusal to acknowledge them and resolve them postpones the inevitable. Eventually, the conflict will blow up, and there will be a big fight. The love-hate cycle will continue.

Often such couples will make up and get back together. But too often they return on the same terms and nothing is resolved. They blow off steam by hating each other for a few days or weeks, and then sweep the problem under the carpet. As long as the conflict goes unresolved, the couple is headed for the same old fight, over the same old issues.

Healthy relationships are a lot like mountain climbing— anything but easy. There are huge obstacles to overcome and sometimes you have to double back and try another route. It's not always easy, but they keep climbing.

Unhealthy relationships are like whirlpools. The love-hate

cycle goes around and around with no real advancement. Ultimately, the relationship goes down the drain.

9. Strengthening vs. Weakening

Addicts feel invincible when they're on drugs. Euphoria reigns. They can do anything, meet any challenge, and conquer the world. The same is true of relationship addicts. When you're with that special person, things are great. When you're in the kind of relationship you crave, you experience a high. When you're engaging in the sexual acts that give you pleasure, or having sex with the person you idolize, the world is yours.

But what about the morning after? What kind of hangover do you have? The sex addict wakes up in a strange bed and feels cheap. The love addict endures the insults or battering of an abusive partner. The person addict sees all of his or her lover's flaws and tries to ignore them once again. The simple question is this: Does the relationship make you stronger? Healthy relationships do. You wake up the next morning and feel better about yourself. You feel empowered by the relationship to try new things and conquer new goals. Addictive relationships sap your strength. The temporary buzz gives way to a lethargic life.

Did you hear that from the people in our circle?

- "I know I should break up with him, but I can't."
- "I really don't believe this is right, but I can't stop seeing him."
- "Every day I tell myself I'm going to break up with him, but then I lose my nerve."
- "I just sat at home and moped."
- "That's just the way I am."
- "I've been trying to break up with him for about six months, but . . . ."

Ironically, the one thing most of these people need to do is to end the relationship. But they simply don't have the strength to do it. Why don't they have the strength to act? That very relationship saps it. For the most part, these women are strong and successful. Some of them thrive in the business world. Others run their households with skill and decisiveness. But these relationships reduce them to children. They think little of themselves. They are afraid of doing something wrong. They have no strength to control their lives.

It's also ironic that the people who are strong enough to stand on their own—even to break off a close relationship—are the ones who don't need to. Healthy relationships give people the kind of support they need to make important decisions, feel confident, communicate freely. And those are the relationships to hold on to.

The Cycle

Addictive relationships follow certain patterns. Some who go from relationship to relationship find themselves doing the same things in each one. Obviously, details may differ from person to person, but here's the general picture.

1. *Initial emptiness.* You're in need. This may be the result of a recent disappointment—a breakup or divorce. Or it may be a general lack of self-esteem, perhaps a result of your upbringing.
2. *The connection.* You meet a person who seems to offer exactly what you need. Perhaps the person singles you out for attention, which pleases you. Or perhaps it's someone you decide to pursue.
3. *Infatuation.* The mind games begin. Infatuation is a normal start to many relationships, but you may go overboard this time. You begin to idolize the person. You think about the person often, remembering only good things, ignoring faults.
4. *Feedback.* At some point, you may have friends giving

you their opinions. They say the relationship is bad for you. But what do they know?

5. *Excuses.* You make all kinds of excuses to yourself and to your friends. It's not as bad as they think—or so you say. You have nagging doubts about the relationship, but it's the best thing that's happened to you in a long time.

6. *The turning.* There's often a point where you commit to the relationship, just within yourself. This is where some people distance themselves from their friends. "If you don't like him, then tough! I don't like you." At this stage, you tire of making excuses. Sometimes you scuttle your convictions about churchgoing, sexual morality, or what you'll put up with.

7. *A step too far.* The relationship may continue for a long time before something happens to jolt you back to your senses. Maybe your partner is unfaithful or abusive. Maybe you finally see how far you've plummeted. There is new dissatisfaction with the relationship.

8. *Panic.* Whenever you think about ending the relationship, you get panicky, sometimes clinging to the person even more. You've invested a great deal of yourself in this relationship. It scares you to think of letting it go. This doublemindedness—bouncing between steps 7 and 8—can continue for months or years.

9. *Breakup.* The relationship may never get to this point. But you may override the panic long enough to make a move to get free of the relationship. In some cases, the other partner initiates the breakup, which causes great pain.

10. *Withdrawal.* After the breakup of an addictive relationship, you can expect to suffer withdrawal symptoms that are not only emotional but physical as well. Your body has grown used to the sensations of that relationship and now must readjust. In addiction, you've probably been

through great tension in making the decision and/or suffered shock when the breakup finally occurred. You feel lousy. What do you do?

11. *Return to sender.* Unfortunately, many people decide that the most obvious way to overcome their withdrawal symptoms is to go back into the relationship. They feel lousy, and going back will make them feel better. Or so they figure. This is, in a sense, another "turning," and they go back to step 6.

12. *New game.* Eventually the relationship ends for good, and you fight through the withdrawal symptoms, but you still feel empty, alone, and lost. If you're smart, you'll restore contact with those friends you rejected around step 5 or 6. But too many go back to step 1. They feel empty, so they seek fulfillment in a new relationship. And the cycle starts all over again.

Recognizing Relationship Addiction

Now that we've covered some of the general characteristics of addictive relationships, the question is: Would you recognize them in yourself if they were there?

Sometimes it's easier to see the weakness in others.

The following letter came to me recently. Read through it and see how many of the addictive characteristics you can spot. Then go back and see if any of it sounds like you.

I'm sitting here writing to you through tears, soliciting your prayers. I've been separated and divorced for three-and-a-half years. I finally allowed myself to fall in love with a man with whom I've had a wonderful relationship for over five months now. We spent a lot of time together and became very close very quickly.

About two months ago, he told me he wanted to marry me. We knew that this was the direction in which we both wanted our relationship to go. Then, out of the blue, he announced that he couldn't go through with this and wants nothing to do with me. He insisted he meant everything he said about love and marriage but really needs to be single for right now. When he told me this, he was very cold, detached, and somewhat hostile. He'd never been this way before.

He told me he had a temper, but I had only seen it a couple of times, and I just figured he was having a tough time emotionally. He told me I was good for him because I brought him closer to God. Before he met me, he was into porno films and occasionally solicited prostitutes. Once he told me he would rape me unless I consented to have sex with him. This may sound crazy to you. But I am an educated person and no dummy! I believed in this man, and I accepted his past as just that. It was in the past! He was a gentleman, and treated me so well. We even prayed together and said grace before every meal. So I obviously believed him and trusted him.

Why do my pastor, his pastor, and my therapist all see this man as a person with a character disorder and a sexual deviant? They tell me to get out of Dodge in a hurry and to count my blessings that he dumped me. None of them know him like I do.

I am emotionally devastated. I trusted, and now WHAM! Where did I go wrong? Now I'm grieving all over again, and this time it's worse than my marriage breakup. I don't know how I will go on without him.

I am probably the first one who ever loved him unconditionally. He even told me I was. Maybe he couldn't handle it. Who knows?

Please pray for me. My self-esteem is shot, and I feel so used. I still believe in my heart that he is a good man at his core. Pray that he will get help, too, before he goes out and does something stupid (for instance, rape).

> Please send me anything you can that will help me.
> I have a lot of love to give to someone. Pray that I will
> find someone soon who can accept that love and who
> can share my same needs and desires.

My purpose is not to judge but to help. By shining the spotlight on this often-ignored subject of relationship addiction, perhaps I'll motivate some readers to get the help they need. Perhaps some friends will sense what kind of help is needed.

The woman who sent this letter did a number of things right. She was praying. God's help is crucial to break an addiction, as any twelve-step program will tell you. She was seeking counsel from pastors, a therapist, and (through this letter) me. She says her self-esteem "is shot," but her letter indicates that a strong sense of self remains. "I allowed myself to fall in love . . . ." "I am probably the first one to love him unconditionally." Although she was confused and hurt, she was not curling up in self-pity and self-hate.

The letter, however, clearly depicts the dangers of codependency. She was trying to rescue this man. She felt she was the only one who could get through to him. He needed her, and she thrived on being needed. (Note that her current frustration is that she has so much love to give, but no one needs it.) Although she was probably much more stable emotionally than he was, she became fixated on him. He became her reason for being. She was bringing him to health, to love, to God.

Also, did you see how many times she contradicted herself? Could you see her rose-colored glasses? "He was a wonderful man. He said he would rape me. . . . He was a gentleman. . . . I trust him, but I'm afraid of what he'll do. . . ."

Why did he break it off? We don't know. It may have been a flare-up of his sexual addiction. Perhaps he didn't want to become healthy—just yet. Perhaps she was smothering him with her zeal for rescuing. Reading between the lines, we might guess that he was not being totally honest with her about his addiction, his temper, his desires.

Relationship addiction is a powerful and dangerous thing. It grabs us at the core of who we are and makes us do things we'd never dream of. The drug addict would betray his own mother for a fix. The compulsive gambler would steal from his best friend in order to place just one more bet. And the person addicted to love would sacrifice principles and friendships and self-respect to go out "just one more time" with that special person.

The first step in any safari is to identify the beast you're hunting. What does it look like? What are its habits? Where does it hang out? We've done this. We now know what addictive relationships look like.

But the next step is to gauge the level of danger. What kind of danger are you in? Are you in an addictive relationship or about to take the plunge? Would your current relationship be considered "addictive"? The next chapter's test will answer some questions for you.

CHAPTER FIVE

Test Yourself

ℱᗩ

Y OU'VE READ ABOUT THE DIFFERENT TYPES OF RELATIONSHIP ADDIC-
tion and nine of its major characteristics. Now it's time to
test yourself. Do you have a relationship addiction, either to a
particular person or to a particular kind of relationship? The
following questions will help you sort that out. While this is
not meant to be a scientific study, it should provide you with
ideas about your general tendencies.

As you can see, your possible responses range in value from
1 (strongly disagree) to 7 (strongly agree). If you are totally
unsure, don't skip the question—just circle 4. Answer as honestly as possible how you feel about each of the sentences presented. And don't try to "psych out" the test. Don't try to figure
out whether it's good or bad to answer a certain way. Some statements are really rather neutral. But, taken together, they will provide helpful insight into your tendencies.

You can mark your answers in this book or you may want
to use a separate piece of paper so you can lend this book to a
friend or perhaps re-test yourself a year or two from now. (You
have permission to photocopy the scoresheet. That's important
for analyzing your responses.)

The Test

Relationship Addiction Test Key

1—Strongly Disagree
2—Disagree Somewhat
3—Lean Toward Disagreeing
4—Neutral/Don't Know
5—Lean Toward Agreeing
6—Agree Somewhat
7—Strongly Agree

---

1. I do not feel happy unless I know that someone loves me.

   1   2   3   4   5   6   7

2. I feel an irresistible impulse to pursue a person I am attracted to.

   1   2   3   4   5   6   7

3. If I think someone really needs me, I am attracted to that person.

   1   2   3   4   5   6   7

4. I do not have the resources within me to deal with the emotional pain I face.

   1   2   3   4   5   6   7

5. When I am not in a steady loving relationship, I feel empty and needy.

   1   2   3   4   5   6   7

6. I sometimes feel guilty about going too far sexually.

   1   2   3   4   5   6   7

7. I can easily identify one person I'm attracted to above all others.

   1   2   3   4   5   6   7

8. My parents had addictive tendencies.

   1   2   3   4   5   6   7

9. I fantasize about an ideal mate who would know me and love me thoroughly.

   1   2   3   4   5   6   7

10. I tend to view each new person I meet (of the opposite sex) as a potential conquest.

   1   2   3   4   5   6   7

11. I tend to ignore the flaws in the person I'm in love with.

   1   2   3   4   5   6   7

12. When I think about my childhood, I have unresolved issues that still cause me pain.

   1   2   3   4   5   6   7

13. I think there's something wrong with me that makes me hard to love.

   1   2   3   4   5   6   7

14. I often feel inadequate sexually.

   1   2   3   4   5   6   7

15. I think I can change the flaws in the person I love.

   1   2   3   4   5   6   7

16. I feel that I usually give in when others want something from me.

   1   2   3   4   5   6   7

17. Sometimes I'm treated unfairly in a relationship, but it's worth it just to be loved.

   1   2   3   4   5   6   7

18. I fantasize about an ideal lover who will give me great pleasure.

   1   2   3   4   5   6   7

19. The person I'm in love with makes up for my shortcomings.

   1   2   3   4   5   6   7

20. My romantic relationships tend to vacillate between love and hate.

   1   2   3   4   5   6   7

21. When I am in a romantic relationship, I tend to let all of my other friendships drift away.

   1   2   3   4   5   6   7

22. I feel most loved when I am involved in sexual intimacy.
    1   2   3   4   5   6   7

23. I get extremely jealous when my partner shows interest in someone else.
    1   2   3   4   5   6   7

24. I have recently suffered an emotional trauma that brought me great pain.
    1   2   3   4   5   6   7

25. When I am in a loving relationship, I feel energized and powerful.
    1   2   3   4   5   6   7

26. I often find myself fantasizing about having sex with people I see on TV or in the movies.
    1   2   3   4   5   6   7

27. I feel physically ill if I have to be away from the one I love for a week or more.
    1   2   3   4   5   6   7

28. When I am in a relationship, it tends to control my life.
    1   2   3   4   5   6   7

Scoring

1	2	3	4
5	6	7	8
9	10	11	12
13	14	15	16
17	18	19	20
21	22	23	24
24	26	27	28
(L)	(S)	(P)	(G)

How to Score

Write the number you circled next to the question number in the table. Then add up the totals for each column and write them next to the appropriate letter: L (Love Addiction), S (Sex Addiction), P (Person Addiction), and G (General Addictive Factors).

Next we'll look at what the scores mean.

Love Addiction (L)

As you recall, love addiction is the compulsion to be in a relationship, the perceived need to be loved. It's often related to low self-esteem. The love addict feels a need to be with someone else in order to "be somebody." The love this kind of addict craves is not really love, but the feeling of being in love.

45-49 You feel like you need a romantic relationship in order to survive. This can get you into trouble as you jump into bad relationships just to be in one. Read this book, but don't stop there. You may need to see a professional counselor.

39-44 You have a strong tendency toward love addiction. You have high expectations for romantic relationships, and probably a low estimation of what you can accomplish on your own. You need to move toward more realistic understandings of both of these areas—and be careful about the relationships you're in.

32-38 You lean toward love addiction. While it may not be an ongoing danger for you, it's something to watch out for, especially if you face a sudden trauma, such as a painful breakup or family crisis. Shore up your own self-esteem—it will help prepare you for any rough times ahead.

25-31 It's not a problem, but be aware of any sudden changes in your attitude, perhaps brought about by a crisis of some kind. Especially if you score high in another area of relationship addiction, you could easily slide into a love addiction as well.

Below 25 You are below average on the danger scale. This doesn't seem to be a problem for you at this time.

Sex Addiction (S)

While other books these days discuss sex addiction in conjunction with pornography and promiscuity, I'm focusing on it within relationships. It may be manifested in those other ways, but how does it affect the relationships such a person is looking for or is presently in? Thus the statements that follow don't focus on behavior but on feelings. They measure a tendency toward sex addiction, rather than the actual playing out of it.

45-49 You are in trouble. You tend to confuse sex with love, and you seek to use others sexually to overcome your own feelings of inadequacy. Besides reading this book, consider connecting with a sexual addiction support group and a professional counselor.

39-44 You have a strong tendency toward sex addiction. You probably love and hate sex at the same time. You feel strong sexual impulses and sometimes try to fight them off. You need to work at defining sex and love as separate forces, and strive to gain a healthy understanding of the opposite sex. Be careful about your present relationship, if you're in one. Avoid temptation.

32-38 You lean toward sex addiction. Be very careful and aware of the messages you take in from TV and movies, the music you listen to, the people you hang around with. Our whole society leans toward sex addiction. Don't let it take you for a ride.

25-31 It's not a problem, but watch for any sudden changes in your attitude, perhaps brought about by a crisis of some kind. Especially if you score high in another area of relationship addiction, you could find yourself in a sex addiction as well.

Below 25 You are below average on the danger scale. This doesn't seem to be a problem for you at this time.

Person Addiction (P)

This addiction differs from the others because it focuses on a specific person. If you currently are not seeing someone special, these statements may have been hard to respond to. Perhaps you thought back to past relationships. If so, it's possible that you scored high here, even if you're not in an addictive relationship. But the high score would still show a tendency toward person addiction.

43-49 You are almost certainly addicted to someone, or you are in extreme danger of falling into a person addiction. You tend to look to this person for salvation, for identity, for purpose in life. Try to establish an identity of your own, apart from this person. You may need the help of a professional counselor to do so.

36-42 You have a strong tendency toward person addiction. You tend to "worship" the person you're involved with—or you feel that this person could not live without you. (Person addiction can go both ways—you need your partner, your partner needs you, you need to be needed, and so on. If your situation is more one-sided, you may not score as high, but you may still have a problem.) You need to look for ways to break away, even subtly, and let both of you exist as independent people.

28-35 You lean toward person addiction. (Because some of the questions measure caretaking, which may not apply in all cases, the score breakdown is lower—28 is an average score but could still indicate a leaning.) Be careful about the relationships you get involved in or how you conduct your present relationship. Keep your eyes open to your partner's faults (and your own), and encourage your partner (and yourself) to make independent decisions from time to time.

23-28 It may not be a problem, but watch for growing dependency in a relationship. Work toward a mutuality, an interdependence in which both partners are strengthened as individuals, even as the two of you grow together.

Below 23 You are below average on the danger scale. This doesn't seem to be a problem for you at this time.

General Addictive Factors (G)

As we will see in chapter 7, the roots of relationship addiction go deep into our experiences growing up and with past relationships. These responses measure the existence of these factors. You may score high and still have few problems with addictions, but that would be rare. This score indicates your general susceptibility to relationship addiction.

45-49 You are a relationship addict waiting to happen (if it hasn't happened already). A number of background and attitude factors are present that could easily lead you into addictive situations. Once again, professional counseling may help you deal with some of these.

39-44 You have a strong tendency toward relationship addiction. You need to work at resolving some of the issues from your childhood or from past relationships that are causing you pain. Especially if you recently had an emotional trauma, take the time to heal. It may be best not to be in a romantic relationship right now.

32-38 You lean toward relationship addiction of some kind. Several key factors are present. If you manage these well, you'll be fine. But be careful about bringing unresolved personal issues into your relationships.

25-31 You do not have significant background or attitude factors that would lead you into a relationship addiction. That does not mean you're scot-free. You may still succumb to momentary pressures.

Below 25 You are below average on the danger scale. This doesn't seem to be a problem for you at this time.

ℬ

OBVIOUSLY, your situation is unique. Use these numbers to get a general sense of your situation, but don't be enslaved by them. The test may break down at some point, or you may be an exception. But if you need help in a certain area, you probably know it already. This test just confirms it. Don't be alarmed if you score high in all areas. This is common. Addictive personalities often have struggles in different areas. Use the findings of this test not to paralyze you with worry, but to spur you to action.

CHAPTER SIX

Case Study: Scott

༄

S COTT IS A CARETAKER. HE TAKES CARE OF OTHERS. HE FEELS FULFILLED when he is helping somebody. It's a good way to be, but it has its pitfalls. It's the classic tale of codependency—if you succeed in nursing someone back to health, you're out of a job.

When Scott first came to me, he was involved in a relationship and had lots of questions about it. It was wonderful; it was terrible. It was making him stronger and weaker. It was delighting him and depressing him. He wasn't sure what to do.

He met Julie "by accident," he says. They were at a church retreat, and she thought he was someone else. They had lunch together, and a long conversation that neither wanted to end. Scott was a leader in the church, affable and dedicated. Julie was a young mother, newly separated from her husband. In Scott, she found a listening ear and a warm heart. She unfolded a story of long-term emotional abuse by her husband. She was very, very needy.

This need attracted Scott like a magnet. As he listened to this troubled soul, he was drawn in. *How can I help? What can I do? How can I save this person from her distress?*

Scott was no stranger to divorce. His parents split up when

he was young, and he knew firsthand the agony of alienation. An experience like that can damage or strengthen a person. Even at a young age, a victim of divorce decides whether to be part of the problem or part of the solution. Scott decided to be part of the solution—and he has been a caretaker ever since.

A Blossoming Relationship

A friendship blossomed between this church leader and this estranged wife. Mother's Day was coming up. So she wouldn't feel neglected, Scott sent flowers anonymously, with a note: "From One Who Understands." Did she know who that one was? Maybe. It was just the attention she needed.

Soon she was inviting him to dinner. She had a comfortable lifestyle, having come from a wealthy family. Scott, a lifelong bachelor with a rather low-paying ministry-related job, appreciated her large, comfortable home. It was something he could get used to.

The dinners became more frequent. Their friendship intensified. Julie shared deep secrets of her life, neglect in her upbringing, and betrayal by many of the men in her life. He was listening, nodding, understanding, caring. Even then, he was aware of a romantic undercurrent. He carried on a running monologue within himself: *This is not good. She's still married. This is tantamount to adultery. This is just not good.*

Friendly hugs turned into goodnight kisses, which yielded to even greater intimacy. She overwhelmed him with her physical and emotional needs. She longed to be held, to be loved, to be sexually intimate with a man she cared about. He tried desperately to cling to his moral convictions.

By this time, Scott was convinced that Julie's marriage was beyond reconciliation. He believed in marriage and didn't want to be a party to her divorce. But she was still technically married, and this bothered him. Any sort of romantic interaction was questionable at best. He kept drawing lines in the sand, and Julie kept pulling him across. She wanted—she "needed"—more of his physical attention to her. This became an issue between them. She had a way of winning arguments, though, and Scott kept easing his principles. "It just snowballed," he says, looking back on it. "As we spent more time together, she desired more intimacy and I just kept compromising, compromising, compromising."

Aware of his own moral struggles, Scott stepped down from his church leadership position before anyone else knew there was a problem. Knowing that his friends would disapprove, Scott wouldn't talk about his relationship with Julie. And as he spent more and more time with her, he withdrew from his broad circle of friends.

While Scott was attracted to Julie's vulnerability, he also saw that she was quite strong and resourceful—when she had to be. Even though she was getting family pressure to go back to her husband, she stood firm against their pressure. This was no easy task, considering the perceived power and wealth of her family.

That combination of strength and weakness was compelling to Scott. Here was a dynamic woman, temporarily wounded by a tragedy. That was all the more reason for Scott to be there for her, to care for her, to restore her to that place of strength.

There was also the sense of "You and me against the world." Cult leaders know that they can cement the dedication of their followers if they portray themselves as gravely misunderstood by the outside world. The same holds true in relationships. If you're the only ones who really understand each other, you will often bind together quickly. Who else can the person turn to?

Scott was burning his bridges behind him, alienating his own friends and spending all his time with Julie. She became his whole world.

The divorce proceedings plodded on for some time, and Scott's relationship with Julie plodded along as well. Every so often, Scott would come to terms with the wrongness of it. He would try to break it off. But she would go crazy. "She was an emotional basket case," he says. "I feared for her life." And so he stayed with her.

Second Thoughts

Scott had a good friend in Colorado, whose opinion he respected. With his support structure eroded at home, Scott consulted his friend to get some perspective on it.

"Why are you in this relationship?" the friend asked.

"I don't know," Scott replied.

"You're telling me it's unhealthy, it's driving you crazy, it's ruining your friendships and your spiritual life. Why don't you just call it quits?"

"I don't know," Scott said. "I just can't."

"There's something else there," the friend said. "There's a reason there somewhere."

What was the mystery reason? Romantics might say that these lovers were meant to be together. It might defy all logic, but go for it! Unfortunately, that thinking gets a lot of people in trouble. It seems to me that the "something else" that held Scott to Julie (and Julie to Scott) was addiction, pure and simple. Julie needed Scott to fill the gaps in her own self that were left by her failed marriage. Scott needed to be needed by Julie. That was where he derived his purpose.

The roller coaster continued. A year and a half into the relationship, Julie called it quits. She was frustrated with the boundaries Scott was placing on their physical intimacy. It was "hurting" her, she said. She needed more.

Here it was, his ticket out—right? But Scott was addicted as much as Julie was. It hurt him to be without her. The idea that she "needed" more than he could give was devastating. He was a failure.

It didn't help when she began to date a wealthy man in the neighborhood. "Mr. Megabucks," Scott calls him, with more than a little resentment. If Julie was trying to hurt Scott, she certainly found the chink in his armor. With his job, Scott could never wine and dine Julie as this other man did. He would be there for her, care for her, listen, and sacrifice his own well-being for her, but he just didn't have that kind of bank account.

Maybe Julie wanted to convince herself she was still worth being wined and dined. Maybe she feared Scott was taking her for granted. Maybe she sincerely wanted to try something new. Whatever the reason, she was back with Scott within a few weeks. And things went on as they had—only Scott may have made a few more compromises.

Personal Stuff

A year later, Scott felt stagnant. He was aware that he had foregone his personal growth in order to attend to Julie's needs. He needed to restore himself. Once again, he tried to break up.

"There are things in me I need to work on," he told her. "This relationship isn't helping either of us. We aren't happy. I need to go and work on my stuff. I have to sort some things out. Maybe then I can come back and we'll be better off."

She couldn't take it. For weeks she cried constantly. She couldn't handle her responsibilities—including caring properly for her young son. When Scott stopped taking her phone calls, she called Scott's mother, begging her to change his mind.

When she got through to Scott, she said, "I can't live without you. I want to help you work through your stuff. We can compromise, maybe cut back on how often we're together. Take the time you need, but don't shut me out of your life."

Scott backed down. And he slipped right back into the routine. Every night at her place for dinner, weekends spent there, then vacations together. He didn't get much chance to work on his stuff. He was a full-fledged addict.

He did take another trip to Colorado, though. Maybe Scott was seeking strength to follow through on a breakup, but his friend tried another tactic. "Why don't you marry her?" the friend asked.

Scott was stunned. Julie's divorce would soon be final, and he had thought about this possibility. But why would his friend be suggesting this?

"Look," the friend explained. "I could tell you to break up once and for all, but would you? From everything you've said to me, sure, you should break up—it's unhealthy. But you're not breaking up with her. You don't really want to. So, if that's the way it is, why don't you marry her? Just get out of this limbo."

Shortly after he returned, the divorce became final. They continued to have some problems. She had some health problems for a time, and that drew them closer. But otherwise they were fighting a lot. She was critical of him. She seemed to be pulling away somewhat. And he wanted her more than ever.

At Christmas he proposed. She turned him down. A week later, she wanted to talk.

"It's over," she said. "I want to be friends with you, but just friends. I hope you're not mad at me."

Mad? Why should he be mad? Try "devastated."

The "just friends" arrangement just made things worse. She still invited him to dinner. She still asked him for help with her son, and work around the house, fixing the car, and so on. And on his birthday she initiated physical intimacy—just like old times.

Was she indicating a desire to restore their relationship, to get back together? No, she insisted. They were still broken up. That was just a momentary impulse. "No," she explained starkly. "My love for you is dead. I'm in a different place now than you are. It was just for fun." Obviously both of them were having trouble redefining this relationship.

Devastation

That's when Scott came to me. This change in the relationship had him utterly confused. He was like the recovering alcoholic working as a bartender, feeding his addiction with touch and smell, though not with taste. Julie seemed oblivious to his plight. She felt sorry for him when she saw his anguish, but there wasn't much she could do—short of reviving the romance.

She had changed. She recovered from her position of extreme need. She didn't need Scott anymore. She wanted to fulfill other needs that Scott couldn't touch. She was truly "in a different place." She was trying to maintain the friendship she enjoyed with Scott, while staying free from a romantic relationship with him. Why couldn't he be happy with that?

Julie was the strong one now. She previously had controlled him with her need. Now she was setting the boundaries of the relationship, and Scott soon realized that he couldn't change them.

"I'm in the midst of trying to accept it," he says now, a few months after the breakup. "If you did an autopsy on me today, you'd open me up and find my heart in a thousand pieces. It feels like every day I'm having a heart attack. I'm not sleeping well, I'm not eating well. Most mornings I lose my breakfast before I go to work. I'm devastated."

Shortly after Scott came to me, I urged him to go cold turkey. By continuing to see Julie, he was prolonging the pain, and in danger of resuming his addiction. He talked with her about it, and they agreed to avoid each other for a time. That "withdrawal" has obviously had a powerful effect on Scott. The physical symptoms alone are frightening, but he will recover.

The emotional and spiritual recovery will take longer.

"I feel like I failed," he says. "Even though we weren't married, I feel like I got divorced from her." Scott still has the gifts that have made him popular in the past, but his self-esteem is shattered. He gave up his support structure, his circle of friends, and now he'll have to try to restore those relationships. For three and a half years he drew his sense of self-worth from his ability to meet Julie's needs. He felt very, very important to her. But now, when she doesn't need him any longer, it's as if the rug has been pulled out from under him. What good is he?

And that intensifies other problems in his life: dissatisfaction with his job, evaluation of his life ambitions, a certain spiritual reordering.

"We were best friends," he says. "We had great communication. And that's the hardest thing about it. I not only lost my lover, I lost my best friend. Right now, when I'm struggling with my own personal issues, that's the hardest thing for me, that my best friend isn't there."

It's hard for Scott to accept, but this is the best thing for him. He needs to find other survival strategies. He needs to find other friends to help him work out these issues. He needs to rebuild his self-esteem through other activities.

"The funny thing is that I wanted out for so long. Every day for a year or more, I would go home at night and say, 'What am I doing? This is ridiculous! I need to get out of this.' Now I'm just amazed that I'm so frustrated. I'm thinking, 'Why am I struggling with this so much? Why does this hurt so much?', I just don't understand why I care so much and why I'm addicted to wanting to be with her."

Evaluation

This is a textbook case of relationship addiction. Many of the characteristics we've discussed in the last chapter are surfacing in this account.

Compulsion. Even when Scott decided that he had to break off this relationship, he couldn't. There was "something else" holding him there.

Attempt to rescue. Scott was a rescuer from the beginning. That's rooted deep in his nature. Perhaps he learned it young, as a child of divorce, wanting desperately to care for his needy parents. This whole relationship started with a note "From One Who Understands." That is Scott's whole gig—he understands and cares for people in need. That's what he does for a living and in his personal life. Julie needed care, and Scott provided it.

Rose-colored glasses. Scott is still speaking of all the good things that Julie did for him, like boosting his self-esteem. The fact is that she has crushed his self-esteem. (I don't mean to attack her in this. She was clawing her way back to emotional health in the wake of her divorce. But Scott would have benefited by keeping his eyes open to the whole reality of that relationship.)

Exclusivity. Scott gave up his many friends—some who disapproved of this relationship, others he just didn't have time for anymore.

Jealousy. Scott was sensitive about his own low earnings, and jealous of men who could take Julie out in style.

Continuing dysfunction. Scott is a child of divorce, and there are some dysfunctional issues in Julie's history. Both were wounded souls continuing the pattern.

Over-dependence. Julie seemed to go through a normal process of divorce recovery. She depended on Scott a great deal to begin with, but gained strength and self-confidence over a few years, with a few relapses. I would suggest that this early dependence was overdone. (That's why I counsel newly divorced people to avoid new romances for about two years: they tend to depend too much on their new partners.)

Scott, on the other hand, depended on Julie for practical matters such as meals and companionship, and for his self-esteem. The practical over-dependence was bad enough—and it made the breakup especially jolting since his whole lifestyle changed—but the emotional dependence was even more dangerous. Scott was defining himself as a need-meeter, specifically as Julie's need-meeter. But as Julie gained health, Scott became obsolete. And when he was no longer needed, he had no more purpose in life.

Love-hate cycle. The ups and downs of this relationship are evident, and typical of an addictive relationship in which the emotional stakes are so high. As Julie went through the bumpy ride of divorce recovery, Scott went along. He was there when she needed him and rejected when she didn't. His situation is not unlike that of a teenager's parent, helping someone to maturity, but often being rejected in the process. It's important for a teenager to learn to live independently, but that usually occurs awkwardly and painfully. The same was true for Julie. At times she needed him desperately, but at other times she needed *not* to need him. That was necessary, but hard for him to take.

Weakening. At the beginning of this relationship, any onlooker would say that Scott was the strong one; Julie was a basket case. But those roles flip-flopped. As Julie regained confidence (thanks partly to Scott), she became the strong one in the relationship, deciding when and how she needed Scott. Now Julie is doing fine, while Scott suffers. She feels sympathy for Scott's pain, but she will not be dragged into it. (That's a good choice; otherwise, the addictive cycle would just continue.)

Scott was clearly weakened by this relationship. And Julie? Was she strengthened? Perhaps. But I would suggest that her healing would have occurred faster if she hadn't been romantically involved with Scott. If Scott had kept his distance, helping her as a friend and minister, he would have had a better effect in her life.

ৡঌ

SCOTT will heal, though the first few months will be tough. He and Julie must go cold turkey, not seeing each other at all, and that's been difficult for them so far. His healing cannot begin until he slams the door on the romance with Julie.

He needs to redefine himself. He can no longer attribute value to himself only when he is meeting someone's need. He needs to bolster his self-esteem. It's great to serve others, but we are valuable people even if no one else wants our services. Scott desperately needs to learn that.

CHAPTER SEVEN

The Roots of Addiction

❧

"WHY DO I DO THIS TO MYSELF?" YOU ASK, STARING INTO YOUR MORN-
ing coffee. The passion that clouded your thinking the
night before has passed, and you examine your life in the clear
light of day.

You've done this before, haven't you? Previous relationships
have shown those same symptoms. Over-involvement. You allow
yourself to think less and less of yourself. You need this relationship, and if you don't have it you'll just die. You have put all your
eggs in this one basket and now the basket's about to drop. Or
the eggs are just rotting there. You feel trapped in a bad relationship or a bad cycle of pursuit. When will you ever learn? You
wouldn't know a healthy relationship if it knocked on your door
with flowers in hand. You sip your coffee to wake up to a new
day that will turn out just like yesterday, only one crank further
on the downward spiral.

"Why do I do this to myself?"

There are reasons. Your addictive tendencies come from
somewhere. And if you can understand their source, perhaps you
can change some basic behaviors and attitudes. Perhaps you can
break out of this prison.

If I were sitting in my den watching TV and noticed a slow steady drip coming from the middle of my ceiling, I could very easily tape up the crack and go on watching my show. But that doesn't solve my problem, though it may temporarily alleviate it. Sooner or later I would experience a similar leak in another part of the room, or in another part of the house.

I might walk upstairs and find a large puddle in the middle of the floor above the middle of my den. I could clean up the puddle and go about my business, assuming that the problem was fixed. But once again, I would be merely fixing a symptom. I would still have to find out what caused the puddle.

Obviously, the real way to solve my problem would be to find the source of the water. To go into the attic, or up on the roof, to find where the water was getting into the house. Only then could I hope to provide a permanent solution to my leak in the den.

So it is with addiction. Stopping the drinking or going on a diet will treat only a symptom of the problem. Dissolving a relationship or moving away might be a good course of action for a person addiction, but the solution doesn't stop there. Chances are, your addictive tendencies will surface in other ways, perhaps in other relationships. We need to go back to the roots of our addiction and seek a permanent solution through treatment of root issues.

In his book *Addicted to Love*, Stephen Arterburn uses the image of water cascading down a mountain. Our addictive tendencies are something like this, he says. If you dam up one path the water takes, it will find another. His point is to show how the different types of addiction are related, and that often a person will stop one addiction only to start another.

But if I could change that picture a bit, maybe we go to the source of that water—say, a mountain lake. And let's build some conduits, with pipes or natural stream beds, and channel that water down the mountain so that it can serve some useful purpose below. It may be a losing battle if we try to dam up one path after another, but if we go to the source, we can alleviate the destruction and make some good things happen.

You get it, don't you? We need to confront our addictive tendencies at the source. And perhaps then we can reverse the destructive patterns and establish new conduits for that energy.

Experience and research have led us to hypothesize several reasons that people tend toward addictive relationships. These can be classified into three general categories:

1. Genetic tendencies
2. Family-of-origin issues
3. Emotional vulnerability

Let's take a closer look at each one of these roots of addiction.

Genetic Tendencies

Scientists differ on this issue, but some have suggested that there is a certain gene that makes a person prone to addiction. Genes may also determine our personalities and preferred style of relating to others. In our circle of eight people struggling with addictive relationships, six of them had alcoholic parents. Is this just a coincidence?

Since leading that group, I've made a conscious effort to inquire about the hereditary backgrounds of all my addictive clients, and my informal research shows that at least eight hundred of them came from some type of family addiction, whether substance abuse, sexual addiction, workaholism, or gambling problems.

Of course my figures hardly make up a scientific study. But they aren't too far off the more formal research cited by the American Medical Association (AMA). Read this news release:

> The biological approach took a big step forward . . . when researchers reported the identification of a specific gene

that may play a key role in some forms of alcoholism as well as other addictions. Of the alcoholics they studied, 77 percent had the identified gene. The discovery, announced by researchers at the University of Texas and UCLA, is a gene linked to the receptors for dopamine, a brain chemical involved in the sensation of pleasure. Such discoveries, scientists say, herald biological markers that may one day make possible early identification of those most at risk of becoming addicted, allowing more effective prevention and treatment.[1]

The "biological approach" mentioned is one side of an ongoing controversy between "nature" and "nurture." This feud underlies several modern issues. While I'm very interested in the continuing biological research, let me say that I find great problems with a completely biological approach to an issue such as addiction.

Here's my gripe: It's easy to use biology as an excuse: "I just couldn't help myself! It's just the way I am!" People can develop a fatalistic approach to their problems: "I'll never defeat it. It's in my genes."

But even with the recent biological research, those are invalid assumptions. Our genes may give us a tendency toward certain behaviors, but we must still choose what to do. In fact, part of healing must include taking full responsibility for our own thoughts and behaviors. Unhealthy relationships are still unhealthy, and you still need to get out of them, even if you have to fight against your own biology.

Even with the biological data, it's still hard to establish a solid cause-and-effect link. For example, if we just take the most common form of addiction, alcohol abuse, we can reason that the alcoholic also neglected his or her children from time to time. Therefore, what caused the daughter to seek unhealthy relationships as an adult—the addictive gene pool or the parental neglect? The best answer is probably: "To some degree, both." We just don't know the degree to which each factor drove her to find relationships to numb the pain of her empty life.

The Medical Evidence

Let's take a closer look at that biological evidence. While it's not conclusive, there is a growing body of research that supports a genetic link for addictions. Most of the research has been done on alcohol and drug abusers, but the literature also mentions common problems with the way addicts handle their feelings, stress, and depression.

Our bodies naturally produce enzymes called *endorphins*, drug-like substances that make us feel good. These are released to the brain on a beautiful spring day or when I sit down to my favorite meal or when I see the person I love. For the addict, however, these hormones may not be released in the same way, and when they are released, there may be less of them. This affects not only the way they metabolize alcohol, but also their ability to control their appetite, their sense of well-being, how they overcome depression, and the levels of their physiological desires.[2] These findings have dramatic implications for the addict. If they're true, they explain why some people struggle so much over drinking, while to others it's no big deal; why one person gives up cigarettes in one day and another agonizes for a lifetime; and why one person finds his or her entire reason for living in an addictive relationship and another maintains a more healthy balance with a partner.

There has to be more than willpower involved. Some very strong people become like infants in the grip of an addictive substance. And it can't be just a matter of making foolish choices. Some very smart people repeat similar mistakes over and over when it comes to matters of the heart. There's apparently some other factor—nature, nurture, or both—that stacks the deck against certain people.

But what is it that determines that one individual will become an alcoholic, another a chronic gambler, and another a love addict?

Our "Drug of Choice"

There is no research indicating a genetic propensity toward any particular type of addiction—yet. Our technology is not that refined, but perhaps someday this too will be determined. While the same underlying motivations, the same search for meaning, the same need to block our pain, and perhaps even similar genetic irregularities may be present in all addicts, our "drugs of choice" may be very different.

Why is it that more men struggle with drug and alcohol addictions, while more women have addictive relationships? Why do men have a greater problem with sexual addiction, when more women are treated for emotional dependencies? There is strong evidence for both sex differences and personality differences when it comes to determining one's drug of choice.

In this regard, I suspect a much stronger interplay between our inherited tendencies and environmental factors. In other words, we may be born with the addictive personality type, but it may be our upbringing, experiences, and personalities that determine the type of addiction we combat.

Our Personality Types

Is there a personality type that's more prone to addictive relationships? I believe there is. That doesn't mean that other people are automatically free from unhealthy relationships. Even the strongest among us are susceptible. But I have seen a greater imbalance among those with dependent personalities. Such people are followers rather than leaders. They love to serve others. They tend to be very nurturing and caring in relationships.

Is this wrong? Is this personality type bad? No, not at all. If that's the way your personality is, that's how God made you—it's not a mistake. But do you need to be more cautious with the kind of relationships you form? Absolutely! In the same way, the natural leaders and "take charge" people among us need to be careful that they don't dominate and manipulate others. They might be susceptible to a power addiction.

The world needs both personality types. Otherwise where would our nurses, counselors, and loyal employees come from? And where would our salespeople, marketing gurus, and corporate presidents come from? Once again, if we just look at the evidence from our original group:

- Dawn is a nurse at our local hospital.
- Margie is a second-grade teacher in a public school.
- Joy is the secretary for her pastor.
- Laurie is an office manager for six salespeople.
- David is studying to be a social worker.
- Ginnie has had a series of clerical jobs and currently is a secretary to a financial advisor.
- And Karen is a clerical worker who was a missionary before her marriage fell apart.

What other personality types form addictive relationships? Besides being nurturing and dependent in relationships, some evidence indicates that these individuals tend to be more self-conscious, self-deficient, and conventional (conforming).

Self-conscious. They are sensitive to criticism and may frequently feel that others don't like them, though they may have no concrete evidence to make that conclusion. They are nervous in public or in the spotlight of attention. They think about themselves a lot, constantly second-guessing themselves. "Should I have said that?" "Maybe I should have done it differently."

To find relief from this self-absorption, such people try to find partners they can pour their lives into. Within these relationships, they attain a certain degree of acceptance and are at least distracted from their self-doubt.

Self-deficient. These people tend to have a low self-image and to struggle with guilt and shame. They feel unworthy around others and therefore seek relationships with those who are considered (by friends and family) "beneath them." They spend much of their relational time trying to prove themselves and measure up to other people's standards. Whenever a relationship fails, they tend to blame themselves and identify some personal weakness.

In extreme cases, they may engage in self-punishment. Putting themselves into self-defeating situations just to prove to themselves that they really are worthless and deserve punishment. This may be unconscious behavior.

Conventional/Conforming. Unlike those who struggle with other types of addictions, the relationship addict tends to be quite conventional and to follow the crowd. This personality trait may be a factor in determining the type of addiction one chooses. Substance abusers tend to be risk takers, unconventional and rebellious, while the relationship addict is very different.[3] The root insecurity of relationship addicts leads them to seek approval rather than escape. To be alone is awful. To stand out in a crowd is shameful. Such people must be part of a group or attached to another person.

If you have one of these personality types, it does not mean you're doomed to addictive relationships. It means you're *susceptible* to them. If you don't fit into these types, it doesn't mean you're not susceptible. It just means you're not as susceptible as those who do fit into these types. There is a complex synergy that leads to relationship addiction. Genetic factors and the personalities we're born with—these just provide a few pieces of the puzzle. For the rest, we need to consult the "nurture" side of things.

Family of Origin Issues

We've made a pretty good case for the theory that our genetic tendencies form the roots of our addiction, but now we need to look at a second factor, which can act just as strongly on us: family background and experiences. What is it about the way we were raised that could cause us to seek unhealthy relationships in our adult life? In general, I've observed that those who struggle with addictive relationships either grew up in a home where they never saw healthy relationships or where there was some type of love deprivation.

Love Deprivation

People can be deprived of proper love and attention for many reasons. Victims of love deprivation include:

1. Children who did not properly bond with one or both parents in their earliest years of life, due to extended hospitalization, foster care, or inconsistent caregivers.
2. Children who bonded early, but then lost contact with either parent or both parents during childhood due to death, separation, or the inability of the parent(s) to care for them. This inability to parent can apply to those who were alcoholic, drug-addicted, mentally ill, extremely dysfunctional, or chronically absent.
3. Children and teens who had little nurturing from one or both parents due to a lack of love, frequent absence, neglect, or abuse.
4. Teens, young adults, and adults who have experienced a lack or loss of love from a series of significant persons in their lives.

In our circle, as the participants discussed their own family backgrounds, we discovered the common thread of alcoholism and dysfunction, as mentioned earlier. But along with this family background came the obvious neglect and sometimes deprivation that go hand-in-hand with specific dysfunctions. Several group members described absent or uncaring fathers they constantly tried to please, though they received very little acknowledgment of their effort. Others spoke of mothers who were cold, distant, or uncaring. Whatever the case, the result was the same. Feeling unloved and uncared for as children led them to seek love desperately as teens or adults.

In our group, David talked about his parents' separation when he was about ten years old and their eventual divorce. But the deprivation began long before Dad's final departure. As far back as he can remember, his mother was in and out of the hospital. Later, as a teen, he found out that her absences were spent at a mental hospital, but as a preschooler he knew only his mother was gone. He was left with babysitters and relatives so his father could work. And even when his mother was home, she was chronically depressed, which meant she had little energy for nurturing her son.

David can't remember a time when he felt secure and consistently loved. Instead, he felt great emotional distance from his mother and abandonment from his father. In adult life, David seeks love wherever he can find it but, as stated earlier, the women he dates never seem to measure up. He is attracted to them, pursues them, but then can't trust the fact that they will love him unconditionally and not abandon him. So he usually rejects them before they have the chance to leave him.

Ginnie's pattern of addiction seems different from that of other group members, but the seeds of addiction are similar. Ginnie described her father as being "unobtainable." He separated from the family several times while Ginnie was growing up, but even when he was home, he didn't pay attention to her. She tried to get his attention by following him around the house, then by asking him lots of questions, and later through her accomplishments at school, but the result was always the same. He wasn't interested in her. Even as a teenager, when Ginnie swore she would not allow him to affect her life, she still found an unquenchable desire to have his approval. Today as a thirty-something adult, she's still seeking his love. She has compensated by finding a way to get other men to notice her. Since high school, Ginnie found that she had a very powerful influence over men—even older men her father's age, such as teachers and neighbors.

Ginnie learned how to dress and act provocatively. She soon

began to act on her sexual impulses, and she found a whole new world of male attention opened up to her. Men not only noticed her, but they began to seek her out and flock around her. This was reassuring, but it didn't last. Each time she thought she found a special relationship, she soon felt the rejection of an unreturned phone call or being stood up for a date. This rejection only made Ginnie even more determined to find acceptance. And she always led with what she thought was her greatest asset. She knew she could appeal to men sexually. It wasn't so much the sex that she was interested in. In fact she claimed that she didn't even enjoy that part of it. She merely wanted the attention, the holding, the affection, the kind words.

Ginnie became good at going to a club or a bar and going home with whomever she chose. When she was out with her girlfriends, she unconsciously competed for the attention of any men who came around—and usually got it. Of course, this alienated many of her friends and drove her even deeper into her empty life of addictive love.

Ginnie and David are very different, but both are examples of those whose parents have imprinted a love deficiency onto their children. This imprint can follow them for the rest of their lives until they find some way to fill the void.

Finding the Love We Crave

It's a simple equation. If we don't get enough love as children, we seek it as adults. The problem might be an absentee father, a distant or uncaring mother, abusive parents, or emotionally neglectful loved ones. In all these cases, children grow up without the proper basis for loving relationships, and without the proper role models of unconditional love. This doesn't always result in unhealthy adult relationships, but that's the tendency.

Sometimes the unmet needs from our childhood drive us to medicate the pain of our empty lives through drugs, alcohol, sex, or gambling. These temporary fixes help for a while, but when they fail us (and they always do), we try something else, perhaps something more socially acceptable: work, food, religion, or a relationship. But we soon find that ultimately no object, no substance, and no relationship has the ability to satisfy the void of an empty life, a life without the security of an unconditional love.

Exploring your family of origin and the pain from your past can be a tedious process. The goal is not to find an excuse for self-pity or even to find someone else to blame. The goal is to figure out what went wrong and then how to fix it. Early childhood imprints make powerful impressions on us. To overcome their influence, we must recognize what was wrong in our childhood, understand how it affects our lives, learn what we can from the experience, and determine to change the future for ourselves and our children.

Emotional Vulnerability

There's a third reason people enter addictive relationships: they're emotionally vulnerable, usually because of some loss or specific need in their life. These people may have grown up in loving homes, with parents who were not alcoholic or addictive, and yet for a period of time they become very susceptible to addictive relationships.

I know firsthand because it happened to me.

I grew up in a loving home where no addiction was present. Other than puppy love in junior and senior high, I would have to classify my love relationships as being fairly healthy. Certainly I had no tendency toward addiction. That is, until I experienced a divorce after four years of marriage. The divorce sent me into an emotional tailspin that lasted at least three years. I felt empty and lost. I actually felt as if part of me were missing, as if I had a gaping hole in my chest. My immediate desire was to find some way—any way—to fill that hole.

Most people believe the best thing for a person who's just had a romantic breakup is to find someone else to love as quickly as possible. How many times have you heard that on TV—or in real life? How many times have you said that?

"What you need now is a hot romance to take your mind off your troubles." Unfortunately, that prescription merely leads to an addictive relationship—one based solely on *my* need for affirmation, *my* emptiness, and *my* desire to be loved again.

In the wake of my divorce, I got involved with a woman who met my needs. Well, actually she met my immediate needs, the needs that were on the surface. She was someone to be with, someone to care for me, someone to cook my meals. And, boy, could she cook!

Our romance was doomed from the start because it was a need-based relationship. It was lopsided. As long as I was hurting, she could nurse me back to health. But as I regained my emotional strength, there was no more basis for the relationship. I believe my recovery stalled for a while as I figured out what to do about this new dependency. (Why get healthy when there's someone here to take care of you?) When we finally did muster the strength to be honest with each other, we broke up amid great pain.

What I needed, and what other emotionally vulnerable people need, is to allow the wounds to heal slowly—to become whole again. Just as a broken arm needs to be put in a cast, so our hearts need to be immobilized so we don't use them again before they are completely healed. And as with that broken arm, if we insist on trying to love again on a broken or wounded heart, it will only hurt all the more. If we continue to try to use it anyway, it's liable to heal crooked.

In our culture, divorce is the most common cause of what you might call catastrophic emotional vulnerability.

I knew a young man who was struggling with dissatisfaction in a dead-end job. He didn't feel significant. There was a young woman he knew who had just been through a divorce, and had two young children. She desperately needed security. You could probably guess what happened. They got together for an on-again, off-again romance that held them in an addictive grip for a couple of years.

He did provide her with some security. It was great for her to know that someone loved her. And she did make him feel significant. But that's about all they did for each other. In many other ways, their affair was unhealthy. They compromised principles, ditched other friendships, and often fought with each other.

There's irony there. Good relationships do provide security and significance. But in our desperate attempt to find these things, we often end up in bad relationships that rob us of these very things. We need balance. It often happens as it did with the couple I just mentioned: one's security is another one's significance. He felt important for being her anchor in tough times. She felt secure because he drew his significance from her. But when she needed to feel more significance, it threatened his. And when he needed security, she couldn't provide it. Their relationship was seriously tilted.

Healthy relationships need to provide both security and significance—and a host of other things. You may have no family history of addiction and your upbringing may be splendid, but a sudden emotional jolt in adulthood can knock you into some bad decisions. Take your time. Heal slowly. And when you are ready to enter a new romance, maintain balance.

CHAPTER EIGHT

Case Study: Bonnie

ℬℑ

B ONNIE CAME TO ME FOR COUNSELING BECAUSE SHE WAS TROUBLED about a dating relationship she just couldn't shake. She knew it was unhealthy but couldn't summon the strength to break it off.

Frequently I find deeper issues in people's lives—ongoing unhealthy patterns. It's like the guy who goes to the doctor with a sore throat and ends up in the hospital for three weeks with some tropical disease. The "presenting problem" is often just the tip of the iceberg. The underlying needs are more titanic. Bonnie was such a case.

"Every relationship I've been in has been a mess," Bonnie told me. "I don't think I've been in a normal one yet." That made me start digging into her history.

She was the middle child in her family. One older brother and an older sister went through school ahead of her and made their marks. They were stars—athletes, scholars, class leaders. Bonnie was ordinary by comparison. And the comparisons were frequently made. "I didn't have a chance," she said, looking back on those days. And her younger sister always seemed to get more attention as the "baby" of the family.

Her great love was music—she sang beautifully—but her parents pressed her to do something more practical. Music was fine for a hobby, but she would have to make a living somehow. Bonnie wished she could apply her talents more, but instead of arguing, she complied with their wishes. Besides, she was sure they knew what was best for her. What could she possibly know? "I had zero self-esteem," she told me.

Round One: Chris

Bonnie went to a Christian college and began to blossom a bit with her new independence. Though she was still rather shy, she dated a number of different men. "If you dated the same person more than a couple of times," she explained, "people would begin to link you romantically with that person." So most guys just dated her a couple of times, then moved on. But then Chris came along.

He was a whirlwind, wining and dining her, showing her attention, showering her with gifts. He wasn't wealthy, but she was his queen. Even in those early dates, there were conflicts. He had a bad temper and would sometimes snap at her. But she tended to excuse these episodes. After all, he was spending so much on her, he had to be in love with her. "Besides," she reasoned, "he was probably the best I could ever get." She had struggled for so long with her self-image that with all this attention, she found herself feeling better than she ever had before. This feeling had to be love. And she knew she wanted more of it.

True, Chris was an authority figure. That was the plan, as Bonnie had learned from her parents' example and from her personal religious views. Men rightfully have authority over their children and over their wives, she believed. If the relationship continued, she knew she would move out from under her father's authority to be under Chris. And Chris was already taking control. Bonnie's parents had some reservations about Chris, but she didn't want to hear them. They caught him in some lies.

Her friends worried about his temper, but Bonnie already felt trapped in this relationship. She married Chris.

Mission Impossible

"He talked me into quitting school and working to put him through," Bonnie told me. "That's how trusting I was. He knew I wanted to be a missionary, so he decided we would be missionaries. For that he would need a degree—I wouldn't."

They decided—well, he decided—they'd work in France, not far from Paris. They were appointed by a mission board for a church-planting project and toured churches to raise support. This was Bonnie's dream. Her brother and sisters had married well and gotten good jobs. But now she was "one-upping" them—she was a missionary, the best job a Christian could have. She feared it was all too good to be true. She was right.

When they got to France, Chris dropped his pretenses. He'd always been a model Christian—in public anyway. He was quick to quote Bible verses and give pious answers. But now he could drop the act. He let Bonnie know he was not interested in serving the Lord at all. He wanted to evade the draft and see the world. She was stunned.

Over the next few years, Chris played a game, sending letters back to their supporting churches with news of how unresponsive the mission field was, while indulging in the Paris night life and developing a pornography addiction. Bonnie was trapped in a foreign country under false pretenses, now pregnant and financially dependent. She felt she had to help cover for him.

Chris tried to appease Bonnie with gifts. They lived in a nice house and drove a nice car, but he was a fraud and now she knew it. "There was no emotion," she told me. "Despite all the gifts, he felt nothing for me."

The dishonesty also bothered her deeply. She was furious at him for his deception, and she felt guilty for joining in deceiving the folks back home. One day she found his briefcase full of pornographic pictures. She taped them to the refrigerator. "There!" she said. "If that's what you want, then there it is! Don't try to hide it!"

And then she found evidence that he was being unfaithful to her. She confronted him with her evidence, but he denied everything. She let it drop. But as evidence and tension mounted, she refused to sleep with him. He stayed in the basement, coming and going as he pleased.

When their three-year term was up, Bonnie insisted that she couldn't go on like this. They would have to resign from the mission board. Chris wanted to continue the charade, but she refused and they returned to the States. Yet Chris never admitted his problems. "He told our supporting churches that I was homesick and had to come back," Bonnie says.

So she bore the blame for Chris's moral failings. It appeared she had made an attempt at this colossal spiritual achievement— being a missionary—but couldn't hack it. Once more, in the eyes of her church and her family, she just didn't measure up.

To top it off, the cloud of a broken marriage was hanging over her. Because of her commitment to her wedding vows, Bonnie tried to live with Chris for as long as possible. But it didn't work. She feared at one point that he was molesting their daughter. Knowing he would deny everything again, she didn't know what to do. She finally separated from Chris, but he still demanded visitation rights. When she talked with her pastor about the molestation, he "freaked out" and was no help. Finally Bonnie contacted a social-service agency that stepped in and stopped the visitation. Chris was upset. With his characteristic temper tantrums, he threatened Bonnie with violence. She moved away.

But she was still officially married to him. Her church didn't believe in divorce, her family didn't believe in divorce, and though it was clear that the whole thing was a bad mistake, Bonnie didn't believe in divorce either. So for another several years she was in limbo—separated, but not divorced.

Her instinct was to go back to her parents, but they insisted she try to make it on her own. So there she was, without a full college education, at a make-ends-meet job she didn't enjoy, caring for a daughter by herself, and having failed (or so she thought) as a wife, as a daughter, as a missionary, as a Christian.

Eventually Chris divorced her; he wanted to get remarried.

Round Two: Steve

About that time, a man in Bonnie's church began showing her attention. After fifteen years of being put down by her husband and even more years of not feeling valued by her family, in his presence she felt like *somebody*. Once again she found someone who would build her self-image.

Steve met some needs in her life. She was weak emotionally. Though her marriage had been all but dissolved for a decade, the divorce was still hard to take. It was a final failure. For all that time she had been praying for Chris's repentance and restoration. Now it would never happen. Anger, frustration, and self-hate boiled within her.

In Steve, Bonnie found a calming influence, a good friend, some new confidence. She was a bit uneasy when the relationship turned romantic. It was too soon, she felt. Besides, she still wasn't sure what she believed about dating again after a divorce. But Steve was persistent, and she craved the attention.

He wasn't wealthy enough to wine and dine her, but he showered her with attention, and that was a commodity she longed for. Steve was a leader in her church, a Sunday school teacher and deacon, so she assured herself that the relationship must be okay.

Steve started to push her for more physical intimacy, far more than she felt was morally acceptable. He was talking about marriage, and seemed especially interested in moving into her spacious home. Suddenly she felt used and disillusioned once again. "He was a fake," she told me, "just interested in meeting his physical and material needs. He didn't really care about me or my daughter." She felt let down. If you can't trust a Sunday school teacher, who *can* you trust?

Bonnie lacked the courage to end the relationship with a face-to-face conversation. She tried, but his calming words seduced her again. "Who knows how long I would have gone on like that?" she confessed later. "But finally, I moved away." She went back to the area where her parents lived. The romance was left behind.

Round Three: Ted

She was back in her parents' neighborhood. They were back in her life. She was their child again, thirty-five years old but now unmarried. "They treated me like a little girl," she said. While she sometimes resented this, she also accepted it. She let them make decisions for her once again.

That was also the way she dealt with men.

Ted was an old schoolmate; his parents were friends of her parents. Back in the old neighborhood, she began to see him around town. She was never all that attracted to him, but he was crazy for her. "He kept coming around," she said as she sat in my office. "I'd say, 'Don't show up tomorrow,' but he would anyway."

On their first date, Ted interrupted her in mid-sentence to walk across the room and kiss her. That may seem romantic for long-time lovers, but on a first date with someone who still hasn't made up her mind about you, that's just rude. And obviously, in his mind, what she was saying was not nearly as important as his romantic agenda. Bonnie was troubled by this, but, true to form, she let it pass without comment. She didn't want to create a conflict.

That's how the relationship progressed. Once again, Bonnie was wined and dined and drawn into a relationship. She loved the attention. Yet she knew this man was all wrong for her. He did not share her spiritual interests. Even when he was trying to be good to her, he was overly persistent and rude. He harassed her.

Once he had her under his spell, the wining and dining degenerated into using and abusing. He would call at the last minute for dates, take her to cheap places, and seem more eager to get physical with her than to talk with her. She found it odd that he never introduced her to his friends, and he often went away for weekends without an explanation. Her friends, her parents, even her daughter were all telling her to dump him, but she didn't know how.

She tried. Eight times she tried. But he kept coming back. And again and again, she fell back into his trap. "I kept thinking, 'Maybe he'll treat me nice again, like he did at the start.' You forget the bad things. I mean he really treats me like dirt now. But I keep thinking that maybe I did something to make him change."

Ted was the reason Bonnie first came to me. She felt powerless to make a break from him. Even during our sessions, she was erratic. She would be furious with him one week, defending him the next. Through her counseling, through some journaling, and through our group sessions, she gradually gained perspective and strength. But she used an old strategy to break up with him for good—she moved away. It was just for the summer, but she had an opportunity to work in another state. She quickly took it. She knew that, from that distance, she could view the relationship more objectively.

Bonnie wrote Ted a stern letter, once and for all ending their romance. He must have sensed how determined she was because he left her alone after that.

About a year later, Bonnie was in her driveway washing her car when Ted drove by. He stopped and honked and waved. She smiled politely and continued washing the car. He stayed there, looking at her, perhaps wondering if she'd come over to talk. She didn't. She was determined to stay there, to keep him from once again controlling her life. It was a test of wills, and she passed. He had no more power over her.

While Ted seems to have lost his sway over Bonnie, that doesn't mean her addictive tendencies are cured. In fact, she admitted to me that she might still be seeing Ted if she hadn't gone away that summer. With continued work, she may be able to overcome these tendencies next time a relationship comes around. But there will be a lot of struggle involved. Her addictive ways are deep-seated; they won't be easy to conquer.

Evaluation

Bonnie felt inferior as a child. She constantly sought her parents' attention. There were no signs of addiction in her family, but perhaps we can trace her addictive tendencies to her longing for love and attention. While this is normal for all children, some seem to have a greater need for attention than others. Some have labeled this "love hunger."

When Bonnie married Chris, it seems she was blinded by her own need for love. Chris gave her attention, and she was a sucker for it. She married a man who seemed giving because of his material generosity, but who turned out to be a big disappointment.

Her second relationship was also a result of her ongoing love hunger. She was still afraid of being alone, but now, added into the formula, was the emotional void left by her divorce. She couldn't risk confronting this man about her difficulties with their relationship, so she just moved away. This is her way of solving a problem without really solving it. In a way it works as a cold-turkey strategy, and I suppose it's better than staying in an unhealthy relationship. She may have learned this coping method as a child, when she learned how to avoid conflict with her parents. Nothing was ever gained by questioning or arguing. Just agree or walk away. She's been walking away ever since.

Bonnie's third relationship was also a combination of childhood love hunger and emotional vulnerability. She succumbed to his persistence because her neediness overwhelmed her rational thinking. After a great deal of struggle, she broke it off in the usual way, by leaving for the summer.

I can't say Bonnie is cured, though at present she is free from the bonds of any particular relationship and is moving forward with her life in a healthier way. She is making her own decisions and working hard to take full responsibility for her future—apart from a man. She still hasn't resolved her need for affirmation. That may last a lifetime. But like any disability, one can learn to live with it and overcome its apparent effects.

Bonnie admits to continued insecurity and would "jump at the chance to be in a relationship." Her lack of personal confidence makes her extremely susceptible to any strong-willed man who comes along. That's why in her more rational moments she reminds herself to be extremely cautious. She has also learned to seek third-party objectivity before moving into anything new.

Others in Bonnie's situation have found that a healthy confrontation once in a while is a big help. While I happen to be a conflict avoider myself, I've found that many times it gets me into more trouble in the long run. From this example we can see that conflict avoiders may find themselves trying to please others so much that they forfeit their own feelings and needs. Breaking these patterns takes commitment and wisdom—the commitment to work at changing your natural tendencies and the wisdom to know the proper balance between confrontation and submission.

Bonnie also needs to come to grips with her past. The wounds of her bad marriage, a manipulative husband, and an eventual divorce are still with her, especially in a religious culture that tends to demote divorced people to second-class status. Her weakened self-image was further eroded by each new failed relationship. These scars are not quickly healed. Exploration of past hurts, renewed self-confidence, and a belief in a more loving and accepting God have gone a long way toward improving Bonnie's chances for a healthy relationship.

CHAPTER NINE

Breaking the Addictive Cycle

೪ৡ

Mᴏsᴛ ᴀᴅᴅɪᴄᴛɪᴏɴ ʀᴇᴄᴏᴠᴇʀʏ ᴘʀᴏɢʀᴀᴍs ɪɴᴄʟᴜᴅᴇ ᴀ sᴛᴇᴘ-ʙʏ-sᴛᴇᴘ approach to overcoming problems in your life. There's wisdom in this. Recovery rarely happens quickly or easily. Changes will not happen overnight. It is a process, sometimes long and arduous, and you have to take one step at a time.

The same applies to the relationship addict. The steps of recovery need to be slow, steady changes toward a more balanced understanding of love and healthier relationships.

I still enjoy the movie *What About Bob?*, probably because it features a psychiatrist, played by Richard Dreyfuss. This character advises his client (Bill Murray) to overcome his fears and anxieties by taking "baby steps."

At the end of the session, Murray shuffles out of the psychiatrist's office, carefully putting one foot in front of the other, mumbling under his breath, "Baby stepsbaby steps to the hallway. Now baby steps toward the elevator. Now I'm taking baby steps onto the elevator." As the elevator doors begin to close, he yells out, "Hey, this really works. I made it!"

Get that picture in your mind. If you are struggling with an addictive relationship, there's hope for you. Just remember that comic image of Bill Murray taking his baby steps through life. Step by step you can break your addiction. Sometimes you'll look up and feel depressed because there's so much further to go. Remember: Baby steps, baby steps. If you take one day at a time, you'll be making progress toward mature, loving relationships.

Step 1: Admit You Have a Problem and that You're in an Addictive Relationship (or Are Prone to Such Relationships)

Just as the alcoholic begins his AA experience by standing up and announcing, "My name is _____ and I'm an alcoholic," you must first admit your addiction or tendency to yourself and then to others.

That's hard, isn't it? Personal secrets and family secrets can keep us tied up emotionally for years. The secret takes on a special power, reinforced with each new moment of silence. But when we demystify the secret by saying it out loud and by telling others, it tends to lose some power almost immediately.

I see this phenomenon in therapy all the time. People come in with secrets. As they begin to open up, the grip that the information had on their lives is released. And the fact that they are admitting their own weaknesses, acknowledging their need for help, is often a major part of the therapeutic battle.

One woman hesitantly told me she'd had an abortion. This was a secret known only to her closest friends. She felt terrible about it, but she explained that her circumstances at the time (which included an addictive relationship with a man) had backed her into a corner. And she had lived with this awful guilt ever since. She had a hard time accepting what she had done and felt choked with emotion. But the mere act of confessing it had a powerful effect. A weight had fallen off her back. She punctured the power of secrecy.

This is true of many incest survivors. Every day, it seems we hear a new story of some public figure confronting sexual abuse in his or her upbringing. In most cases, these abuses have been shrouded in secrecy for decades, even blocked within the minds of the victims themselves. But when the secret comes out, the past can be dealt with, and a new future unfolds.

In the case of addictions, the secrecy can be even more difficult to overcome. It's a matter of personal weakness, and that's always hard to admit. The addict needs to say, "This thing has power over me, and I haven't been able to kick it. I've been defeated. I continue to do destructive things." That's hard to say, but it's necessary. It breaks the back of denial.

Denial is the first line of defense for any addiction. "Problem? What problem?" If you pretend it's not a problem, it goes on indefinitely. The first step is admitting it to yourself. You face up to a situation that needs to be corrected. A doctor must diagnose an illness before healing it. This admission is your diagnosis: "I have a problem."

But publicly admitting your problem is crucial, too. For one thing, it keeps you from slipping back into denial. When I say "publicly," I'm referring to telling one or two trusted friends or some type of support group. I'm not talking about putting an announcement in your community newspaper. Once your friends learn you have a problem, the secret is out. It's no use hiding it from yourself anymore.

Emotional support is another result of public admission. You can find power in knowing that there are others who have faced or are facing similar problems. People often fear that they'll be rejected when they finally let their secrets out. But within the right circle of friends, they frequently find acceptance and love. And that can set in motion a whole system of practical support and accountability.

One woman explained to a group of friends that she was mustering up the courage to end a bad relationship. Before the evening was up, one member of that group offered her a place to stay if she needed it, another offered to stay with her, and others offered to be "on call" if she needed someone to talk to, day or night. She had ventured to share her need, and she was met, not with rejection, but with practical assistance. She also knew that she was now accountable to these people, though they had not pressured her at all. She needed to go ahead with this difficult but necessary breakup.

So the first general step toward healing is an admission of the nature of the addictive relationship. Admit it to yourself, admit it to your friends, admit it to the other person in the relationship. If you're not currently in an addictive relationship, but you recognize a tendency in that direction, admit this to yourself and to some close friends. This will help you to be careful when entering a new romance.

Step 2: Recognize that You Can't Change Yourself

Once you've admitted your problem, what do you do about it? Maybe in some cases you could grit your teeth and do what it takes to get whole again and to redeem your relationship. But if you could do that, you probably would have done it by now.

This is the second great lie addicts tell themselves. The first is "What problem?" The second is "I can kick this habit anytime I want." It is the second prong of denial.

In the clear light of day, a woman in an addictive romance may admit, "This is not a healthy relationship." She may even say, "I need to break up with him." But as the sun sets, her old compulsions return. She thinks about him. She needs to see him. She calls him. She goes to see him. And she wakes up the next morning feeling used, perhaps abused, hating herself. "This is not a healthy relationship," she says. "But I can break up with him anytime I want." Right.

How many of these cycles does it take before you realize that you can't? You are held in the power of an addiction that's bigger than you are. You need help.

The Twelve Steps of Alcoholics Anonymous include a reliance on a "Higher Power." Many of us call this power God. We have seen how God changes lives. We have seen how people find strength in a relationship with God. I've been involved with Fresh Start seminars for divorce recovery, where I've seen countless people with deep relational needs—and deep spiritual needs as well. Healing happens on both fronts. As they find God, they tap into divine power to restore their relationships.

It's no magic elixir. It's no "Just trust God and all your problems will go away" kind of thing. But the One who made us has the power to *remake* us. We can rely on Him for the strength we need to restore our relationships and ourselves. Skeptics will say that this is just substituting one addiction for another. In fact, they might say that religion is just another form of relationship addiction, but it's a relationship with God.

It is true that religion can be addicting. You can be drawn to the forms and activities in a self-demeaning and self-destructive way. But there's nothing self-destructive about a true relationship with God. He restores us to wholeness; He builds us up.

As I mentioned in chapter 1, addiction is idolatry. It's a matter of seeking ultimate fulfillment in something or someone that doesn't deliver. We make a god out of some substance, activity, or person. These are false gods—they can never live up to our expectations. As a Christian, I believe that God is the only One who consistently delivers. When God is given top priority, other aspects of life fall into place. But when we allow other substances or actions or people to take His place, we are not whole.

So if you are currently struggling to break free from an addictive relationship, help comes when you look beyond yourself to God. Stop relying on your own power. Ask for His help.

Step 3: Stop Relying on the "Drug"

Just as the drug addict or alcoholic must go cold turkey to unhook from his or her drug of choice, so the relationship addict must abandon the relationship along with any hopes of salvaging even a part of it. (Unless you're in an addictive marriage. There's a special chapter for you later.)

One of the greatest pitfalls I've observed for relationship addicts is their belief that they can maintain some part of the relationship or at least "stay friends." For most people, this might seem only logical, but for the relationship addict, it's disastrous. It's like telling a substance abuser it's okay to drink on weekends or to use cocaine on Christmas and his birthday. Obviously that would be ridiculous advice. It would only lead to relapse.

Relationship addicts often relapse. Why? Because relationships are natural and necessary. It is socially acceptable to be in relationships—and often unacceptable not to be in one.

What do most friends say to someone who's just been through a painful breakup? "What you need is a new romance." No! That's the *last* thing he or she needs. Even if it's not an addictive situation, the post-breakup time requires personal healing, not new love interests. In the case of a relationship addict, the "rebound" can be devastating.

Many times, people try to end an addictive relationship in a gradual way—"to make it easier for both of us." This rationalization only prolongs the agony for weeks, months, or even years. Most of the people I've known who tried this method ended up in a limbo relationship that dragged on until the other person finally called it quits. This can send you into an absolute tailspin.

We saw this in Scott's case. His romance with Julie was addictive, and he sensed it. Though they met some of each other's needs, there was an unhealthy quality to their interaction. Scott felt he needed to break it off—but he didn't. He tried—but always came back. She would call, "needing" him, and he would scurry back to her.

There came a time when she didn't need him anymore. She grew beyond her traumas and wanted to spread her wings a little, so Julie broke up with him. This was devastating for Scott, as you can imagine. The pain struck him physically as well as emotionally.

Yet, amazingly, even after their final breakup, they were getting together "as friends." She felt guilty about dumping him and wanted to salve his wounds. Even in this process, they were still flirting with romantic involvement. They were still addicted to each other, though she had established different terms for the relationship. You may be thinking, "It's nice to remain friends with people you've dated." This may be true with certain relationships or years after the fact, but it's dangerous for those with unhealthy addictions. Scott was pained and confused during this time. Julie was hurting him in ways she never realized.

I finally suggested to both of them that they avoid each other. This was somewhat difficult since they went to the same church. But I asked them to sit on different sides. They needed a clean break so that the healing could begin.

Don't try to kid yourself. As with any other addiction, an addictive relationship must be stopped completely. Immediately. For good. This is particularly true if it is an affair with a married person, or if the relationship is destructive to you or your children. End it *today*.

Step 4: Find Support and Accountability

Let's say you've mustered the strength to end the relationship. It took all you had, but you did it, and now you're free. Congratulations!

But what happens a few hours later, when the adrenaline subsides? When you eat dinner alone or go to a movie alone or sleep alone? Instinctively, you reach for that person you've grown accustomed to. That person isn't there. You feel an emptiness inside.

Do you reach for the phone and call your former lover to patch things up? No. Once again, you grab the strength you need, and you withstand that temptation.

A few days pass. People are asking about your "better half." That's how you feel. Half. You explain things to your closest friends, and let the others draw their own conclusions. You get to the weekend. No dates. Munching popcorn in front of the TV, you remember the joys of weekends past with your ex-lover. Somehow the bad times have vanished from your memory. "Maybe my ex would still take me back," you muse.

It's your birthday. Or maybe your ex's birthday. Or Christmas. A special time, and you're alone again. How will you ever get through? Day after day you fight the urge to run back, to turn back the clock, to climb back into that old relationship. That emptiness still gnaws at you.

And what happens, somewhere during that tortuous process, when your ex-lover calls you? "Let's get together and talk. Just as friends. We need to talk." You're a pushover. The trap door opens. You fall through.

In the wake of a breakup, the pressure to get back together is enormous. It can build through the first few hours of the break-up to a mighty crescendo of emotional despair over the next several months. I have found few who could survive this withdrawal on their own.

What is missing from the scenario I just presented? A support group. Or at least a friend who can hold you accountable to your decision. You need a "sponsor," as many in the recovery movement have called such a person. This must be a person or a group of people who have regular contact with you and who will not accept your first response to "How are you doing?" They must be willing to probe well beneath the surface.

The right group of friends can fill some of the emptiness you feel. They can eat popcorn with you on Saturday nights. And they can monitor your emotions. When you're in danger of slipping back, they can warn you. They will never be able to make your decisions for you, but they can help you see things objectively.

One of the most helpful things that friends do in these cases is to remind you of the bad times. As you look back on an addictive relationship, often you only remember the highs. The lows disappear. Friends are there to tell you what a jerk the other person was, how miserable you were, and how lucky you are to be free.

Tragically, addictive relationships tend to exclude other friends. It may be that a jealous lover forces you to dissolve old friendships, or you may just be so enthralled with your lover that you forget about everyone else. The problem is, these are the very times when you need a circle of close friends. They help you keep your perspective. If your lover is crossing your boundaries, your friends can tell you. They also help you keep a sense of "you." You remain a well-rounded person because you are not totally consumed by your lover.

If you already have a circle of friends to do these things for you, great! But perhaps you have alienated old friends and failed to make new ones. You may need to build new friendships, perhaps among your family or casual acquaintances, or to restore old ones. If nothing else, find friends in community or church groups, or find a counselor who can connect you with an area support group. Much like AA groups, there are sex- and love-addiction groups all across the country. This may be a manufactured support system, but it's better than nothing—and it might grow into genuine friendship.

In any case, you need to empower your friends to support you. That is, you have to *tell them you want them to check up on you.* Among our unwritten rules in this society is: "Live and let live." Many people will consider it rude to pry too deeply into your business—unless you ask them to. If you need their support, say so. If you need their advice, ask for it. If you need their warnings and challenges and scoldings, let them know. You'll probably need all of the above.

Step 5: Keep a Journal of Your Feelings and Progress

If you don't have friends who remind you of the "bad old days," you can do this for yourself by keeping a journal. This is especially helpful if you're in the middle of an addictive relationship.

Start now. Record the good experiences and the bad. Record how you feel each day. Be brutally honest with yourself.

Then, from time to time as you struggle with the relationship, go back and reread the journal. It will give you a sense of your own relational history.

Are you having the same struggles you had a year or two ago? Are you making the same promises to yourself? ("If he or she doesn't shape up in three months, I'm out of here!") If so, that should tell you something. You're stuck.

Or have you sunk deeper into an unhealthy relationship? Are you more attached to the other person than you used to be? Are you more dependent? How has the relationship been unhealthy for you over the years? As you read your journal again, do you like what you're reading? Are you flattered by the picture it gives of you, the writer? Or are there bad priorities, twisted logic, a weak will?

Idealization is a major problem I run into again and again with people I counsel. It's the old rose-colored-glasses routine. I usually have such people go back and read aloud from their journals. It's often a poignant testimony about a troubled relationship—sleepless nights, neglect, abuse. After only a few pages, the reality of the destructiveness of the relationship comes crashing back.

If you're in a bad relationship, journaling can be a way of saving up the ammunition you'll need to get out of it. Not ammunition to attack the other person, but to bolster you in your resolve to get free. If you have already broken free, go back and find those scraps of journaling you may have done earlier—a diary, letters to friends, and so on. Remember how it really was.

Step 6: Understand Your Addictive Cycle and Learn to Control It

Most people have a point of no return. That is, a point at which all reason goes out the window and they decide to go with their emotions. For the relationship addict, that point is dangerous. Picture yourself at the top of a steep hill—on roller skates. As you skate around the hilltop, you have some control over your motion, but when you go too far over the edge . . . well, it's downhill from there.

If you're a relationship addict with a tendency toward unhealthy affairs, it's crucial to learn where your point of no return is. While you're still skating around the hilltop, establish good habits and make wise decisions (take off those skates!). Don't wait until you're in your descent.

The alcoholic learns that he can't go into a bar. There may be nothing wrong with just being there, but he knows that he can't take the temptation, so he avoids it entirely. The drug addict learns that she cannot hang around with the old crowd. They would start pulling her down that slope.

In the same way, the relationship addict needs to learn the triggers for those old, dysfunctional patterns of relating. These triggers may include:

- Holidays, birthdays, or special anniversary dates
- Meeting someone new and falling head over heels in love
- Sensing that someone really needs you
- Feeling undervalued at your job or with your family
- A major loss or crisis
- Any time you feel especially lonely or depressed

You must recognize these as dangerous situations and guard your decisions accordingly. Your emotions must be on red alert at these times. Don't make rash commitments. Take your time. Think things through. Get outside feedback.

Besides finding your trigger points, you need to find some safe havens. This is the time to get a group of friends together or perhaps just to have one or two friends who are "on call" for you. Maybe there's an activity you can sink yourself into for a while or just a way of talking yourself through the crisis. On more serious occasions, you could consult a pastor or counselor.

The idea is preventive maintenance. Be aware of your red-flag times, and do what you need to do to get through them.

Step 7: Examine Your Self-Worth and Identity

Where do you find fulfillment? What makes you feel most like yourself? When do you feel important? Who are you, really?

These questions strike at the root of our sense of self. And that's precisely where most of us get into trouble with addictive relationships. I grab onto someone else because I need to feel fulfilled. For some romance addicts, it doesn't matter who it is, they just need someone to be in love with. For some sex addicts, it doesn't matter either; they just need someone to be in bed with. If they aren't in a relationship—romantic or sexual—they just aren't themselves.

A friend called me and told me about her new boyfriend. She was bothered because she found herself clinging desperately to him, terrified that he would leave her. My friend was a professional actress who was finding it hard to get work. This romance was the highlight of her life, and she didn't want to let go of it.

Always the counselor, I asked her questions about the relationship and about her life. She was full of praise for her boyfriend and full of complaints about her other friends, her family, and her attempts to get work. "When you're with him, you feel like you're worth something," I suggested. "And when you're not with him, you feel like garbage. Right?"

"Exactly," she said, her voice showing amazement. "How did you know?"

Talk to relationship addicts long enough and you hear patterns in their speech that betray certain ways of thinking.

"I just couldn't live without her."

"He makes me feel like I'm somebody."

"When I'm with her, I don't care what anyone else says."

"When I'm with him, I don't have to worry about anything."

"Before I met her, I was a mess."

"Who am I? I'm John's wife."

Let me say that there's nothing wrong with these statements per se. But listen to them carefully, and you'll hear some underlying problems. The one who "couldn't live" without his girlfriend is implying that he has no life of his own. It's great if he makes you feel "like somebody," but would you be somebody if he weren't around? Of course you would! It may be a nice romantic fantasy to forget about the rest of the world when you're with that special someone, but you are still a member of the human race, with all the accompanying responsibilities. It may be true that your lover pulled you out of a "mess," but does that mean that your life will always be a mess without this person? Yes, you are John's wife, but you are much, much more.

In general, people in addictive relationships don't like themselves very much. They long for someone to take them out of themselves or somehow to fulfill them, save them, make them worthy. If you're in an addictive relationship or have that tendency, you probably know what I'm talking about. You're either seeking to prove yourself or to lose yourself. Neither is healthy.

Recovery requires that you first examine your assumptions about yourself. You may already know that you have a poor self-image—or it may surprise you. David, from our original circle, thought he had a great self-image. But as he examined his assumptions, he realized that he had always felt inadequate with women. His addiction to the conquest of women stemmed from that inadequacy; he kept trying to prove himself worthy. There are many overachieving women, strong and confident in the workplace, who subconsciously see every romance as a way of proving themselves to distant or alcoholic fathers.

What do you *really* think of yourself? That's a crucial question to consider.

Once you're in touch with your self-image, what do you do then? Get real. Take a realistic look at yourself—apart from any relationship you're in. What kind of person are you? Are you really as inadequate as you fear? What are your strong points? What people find you valuable, and why? Consult friends or counselors to get outside opinions.

Then talk to yourself. You may think that talking to yourself is corny, but it works. Tell yourself that you're important, that you're a valuable person, even enjoyable. Learn to like yourself. Praise yourself when you do something well. (And hang around others who praise you rather than put you down.) If nothing else, find a simple phrase to repeat to yourself when you begin to doubt your own worth. Something like: "I am created by God and loved by God and others. I am worth something."

If you become more satisfied with yourself, you won't need to seek your identity in someone else.

Step 8: See a Counselor

If the addictive cycle continues to be a problem for you, seek more intensive counseling with a therapist who can help you understand and overcome your addictive patterns. Counseling is not just for crazy people or mental patients. In some ways we can all benefit from counseling, especially if we find healthy relationships elusive. All of us have certain blind spots about our own behavior and attitudes. Counseling will not solve all of your problems, but it's designed to give you insights into why you behave the way you do, and to give you steps to overcome some of your unhealthy patterns.

Counseling provides not only a sounding board, but another layer of accountability. It sometimes helps to have someone to answer to—especially a professional authority figure. If nothing else, you'll want to be sure to get your money's worth, so you'd better get healthy!

ॐ

THE general guidelines of these eight steps will help you break free of addictive relationships and/or stay free of them. The next chapter presents more specific recommendations for people at various points in the addictive cycle.

Chapter Ten

The Slope

A GROUP OF CHILDREN WENT ON A FIELD TRIP TO A NATIONAL PARK. FOR safety's sake (or so they thought), each child had a partner, so no one would be lost. A rope was looped around each partner's waist, with an arm's length of rope between them.

They went to one particularly scenic canyon, and stood on the edge peering down at the stream below. "Be careful, children!" the teacher shouted. "Don't go too close to the edge." Of course, several children immediately went too close to the edge. There they began to play, spinning around, winding themselves up in the rope.

Annie and Barry lost their footing. They began to slide down the edge of the canyon. Luckily, they grabbed at some rocks and stopped their descent just a few yards down.

The teacher hurried to the scene and coached them: "Stay calm. Don't move suddenly. Try to get untangled from the rope. Good. Now Barry, help Annie get over to that rock on your right. Good. Now Annie, pull Barry over with you."

In fifteen painstaking minutes, the children climbed back and were pulled to safety. But a few pairs of kids were oblivious to those events. They were a stone's throw away, doing the same shenanigans that had gotten Annie and Barry in their mess. Cindy and Dan got so wrapped up that they could not move their arms.

"Look, I'm a mummy!" yelled Cindy, her skinny arms tight to her sides.

"Then I'm the daddy!" yelled Dan, bound next to her.

Sarah tugged at her rope. "Come on, Frank. Let's do what they're doing!"

Frank hesitated. "I suppose if they jump into a lake, we have to do that, too."

But, tossing her curly blond hair, Sarah was already winding herself up in the rope and circling Frank.

In their revelry, they hardly noticed the rocks at their feet giving way. All four plummeted into the canyon, helpless to do anything. They got to the bottom, bruised but alive. They cried. They yelled at each other. They worried about what might happen.

"I can't move," said Dan.

"Why not?" Cindy asked, frightened. "Are you paralyzed?"

"No, I think it's just the rope."

"Maybe we could unwind it."

"I don't know," Dan answered. "That seems like an awful lot of work."

Sarah and Frank had fallen a short distance away from the other pair. They too discovered that the rope was hindering their movement.

"Let's get untangled, Sarah. It'll be dark soon and I heard there are bears around here."

"Do you always believe everything you hear?" Sarah taunted.

"Everything except what you tell me," Frank retorted. "It's true. A park ranger told me."

"Oh."

"You got us into this, Sarah," Frank said sternly, tugging at the ropes. "Now help me get us out."

"Can't we keep the rope on?" Sarah wondered. "You're just going to run away and leave me for the bears."

"It would serve you right."

By now, the teacher had a loudspeaker and was calling to the fallen children. "We are sending help, children, but it's getting dark. You must help us help you. First, you have to unwind the ropes. Then you'll be able to move freely. You have to climb out the other side of the canyon. It's not as steep there, and there are signs marking the trail. The park rangers will meet you on the other side. Go quickly, children, while there's still light!"

"I'm afraid," said Dan.

"So am I," Cindy responded.

"I don't think we can get out of these ropes, Cindy. Maybe we can just crawl back up the hill together."

"But the teacher said to go the other way."

"Yeah, but we're right here. Look, it's closer this way. Maybe we can climb back up."

"Okay, let's try it."

They struggled together and moved a few feet. It was too tiring, especially with their bruises. They stopped.

"We'll never get out," Dan whimpered. "We'll just be eaten by the alligators."

"Alligators?" asked Cindy.

Meanwhile, Frank was furiously trying to extricate himself from the rope. Furiously, indeed, since Sarah was doing everything she could to thwart him.

"Don't leave me!" she whined.

"I don't want to leave you, Sarah!" he barked. "But we can't go anywhere like this. It's best for us both if we get untangled—"

"No! You're going to run away and leave me for the bears."

"I'm sure you can manage, Goldilocks."

The teacher periodically called instructions from above. "See that tall pine tree just across the stream? Head for that. The stream is shallow there, and that's where the trail is. Move quickly, children. It's getting dark!"

Every few minutes, Dan and Cindy would struggle a few more feet, but they weren't getting far. And they refused to undo the rope.

Frank, on the other hand, succeeded in getting untangled. But Sarah was being obstinate.

"Will you move your arm, stupid, so I can get this rope off of you?"

"Don't call me that."

"What? Stupid? Well then don't be so stupid and I won't call you that."

"I'm not being stupid. I just don't want you to run away."

"I'm not running away, Sarah. Look, I'm untangling your rope. Does this look like I'm running away?"

"You're just trying to be nice. But when I'm untangled, then you'll run away."

"And you can run with me."

"I'm not as fast as you."

"I'll run slower."

"You will not. Boys never run slow."

"I will, Sarah, I promise."

"Will not."

"Will you just move your stupid arm?"

"My arm is not stupid!"

Frank stopped and glared at his partner. "It's going to be broken if you don't move it."

Sarah moved her arm. Frank pulled the rope around her and found another snag.

"Now lift your foot, Sarah."

"You don't like me, do you?"

"Sure I like you. Lift your foot."

"You'd rather be tied up with Marcie, wouldn't you?"

"Marcie would be lifting her foot right now."

"I knew you liked her. That's why you're leaving me to the bears."

Frank stopped again and wiped his forehead with his wrist. "To be honest, Sarah, I don't think the bears would want you."

"I knew it. You hate me. You're going to run away." Frank

handed Sarah the portion of rope he had untangled. "Here, you try it. I'm going to run and get help. I'll send them back for you."

"I knew it."

He darted off toward the tall tree across the stream. As he went, he heard Sarah's plaintive voice crying, "Here I am, bears! Come and get me!"

Frank's ascent was difficult. He slipped while fording the stream, and got all wet, but he reached the tree and saw the signs marking the trail. He had to stop several times on the climb. When he did, he heard occasional wails from Sarah in the canyon below. He thought about going back to her. Even if he did reach the top, the rangers would never get to her before dark. And if there really were bears. . . .

Once he even turned around and headed back toward Sarah, but then he remembered their argument. Even if he did go back, he figured, he would never get her untangled. So he plodded up the hill again.

Soon he heard voices. Rangers. He called out and they answered. Around the bend and they were there, their flashlights dancing in the darkening wood. Frank told them where he had left Sarah, and where he thought Cindy and Dan had fallen, and several rangers rushed downward while one carried him up the hill.

You can make up your own ending to this story. Frank made it to safety by untangling himself. Were the others eaten by bears or alligators? You make the call.

We have talked about addiction as a cycle, something that's repeated again and again with tragic results in the lives of its victims. Relationship addiction can also be viewed as a slope. You can stand at the crest, teeter on the edge, plummet down the side, wallow at the bottom, or climb out the other side.

This image helps us as we talk about recovery. The solutions are different for those at different spots of this slope. In the early stages of relationship addiction, you can still retreat. You can come back to the top of the slope where the footing is safer.

It is possible that some relationships teetering on the edge of addiction can be saved. Annie and Barry, in the parable just told, are the picture of this situation. They didn't fall far and were able to get back to safety.

But once you're in, once you've fallen into the canyon, the only way out is through and up the other side. There was no way Cindy and Dan could climb back up the slope they had fallen down. Recovery, at this point, requires ditching the relationship and finding personal healing on your own. Frank could have argued with Sarah all night, but it wouldn't have helped either of them. His disentanglement brought the possibility of deliverance for both of them.

Of course the road to wholeness is not easy. The way out of Addiction Canyon is steep and tedious, but step by step you can make it—if you don't look back.

Obviously, that's the most difficult thing about an addictive relationship: breaking up. People keep wondering, "Can't we just do things to make it less addictive? Can't we stay together and just give each other more space?" The answer is no—if the relationship is deeply addictive. There is no climbing back up that slope once you've hit bottom.

I need to mention one exception to this rule: marriage. I don't recommend that those in addictive marriages "ditch the relationship" and go it alone. They have the difficult task of restoring the health of their relationship, honoring their marriage vows. (More on this in chapter 16.)

Let me go on and prescribe specific courses of action for those at different points on this slope (see figure 1). I will be taking the general steps of the last chapter and applying them to specific situations.

1. When You're Not in a Relationship, but Have a Tendency Toward Addictive Relationships

Build your own sense of self. Some people, when they're not in a relationship, spend most of their time whining about

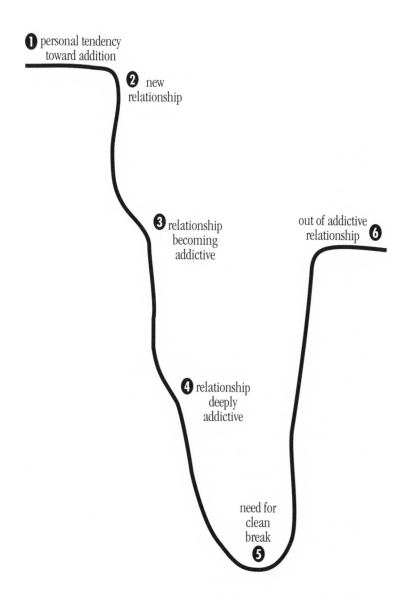

Figure 1. Points sliding into and climbing out of Addiction Canyon.

that fact. It's better to use this time to get to know yourself better. Learn to enjoy your own company. Fill your empty weekends with group activities, special projects, warm baths, and good reading.

Find the things you're good at and do those. Or find something you'd like to be good at and learn to do that. The down time in your romantic life can be a great opportunity to figure out who you really are and to remind yourself of your intrinsic value.

Examine your assumptions.

"If I was worth anything, I'd be dating someone."

"Another Saturday night alone. Nobody loves me."

"I have so much to offer! If no one asks me out, all of that goes to waste!"

"Look at her—one boyfriend after another. She is so lucky!"

"What a babe! Life would be so great if she were my girl-friend!"

"Friendship is nice, but if he really cared about me, he'd ask me out."

All of these assumptions are faulty. But they're common among those who aren't in romantic relationships. Our society attaches gargantuan importance to dating, marriage and sex. The assumptions listed above are reinforced by the media and in everyday conversations. We assume that people who are "with someone" are happy, and those who aren't, aren't.

Take a good look at your assumptions. When you start to say something about the value of being with someone else (or the tragedy of being alone), stop yourself and think about it first. Bad assumptions lead to bad decisions.

See the wholeness in yourself and others. Relationship addiction often arises from a feeling of emptiness. "If only I were attached to that person," you say, "then I would be complete." That's nonsense, of course, but that's the prevailing attitude. And when you say that, you're doing two negative things: you're demeaning yourself and you're demeaning the other person.

You are first ignoring the fact that you're a valuable person in your own right, complete within yourself. By relying on the other person for wholeness, you're putting pressure on the relationship and abdicating your responsibility for yourself.

Second, you're defining the other person as your need-meeter. That person has value to you only as he or she meets your needs. You may "need" someone to be with on Saturday nights or someone to parade before your friends. You may "need" someone to put you through med school or someone to bear (or sire) your children. You may "need" someone to provide for you, share the bills, balance the checkbook, or give you backrubs. But as soon as you begin to define that person by how they meet your need, you're in trouble.

It's common for men who are battling sexual addiction to view women as objects for their lust. Women are reduced to pretty faces and shapely bodies; they are not seen as whole people. (Increasingly, women are viewing men this way, too.) Romance addicts may build fantasies based on one small detail about a person. They think they are loving that person, but they are actually worshiping an image based on merely part of that person.

Fight this. Work to see the wholeness in everyone you meet. When you see people with pretty faces or shapely bodies, ask about their families or any good books they've read lately. Find their flaws and accept them. See them as complete people, even as you remind yourself of your own wholeness.

2. When You're Beginning a New Relationship, and You Recognize that You Have a General Tendency Toward Addictive Relationships

Go slowly. Let the relationship grow slowly. It's not a bad idea to set limits on how often you see each other or talk on the phone—perhaps no more than one date or two phone calls a week. Some have suggested dating several people casually at the same time, though this too can create problems.

The early stages of a relationship set patterns that will be followed throughout the relationship. People with addictive tendencies often rush headlong into new romances, creating unhealthy patterns of relating. Many potentially good relationships are sabotaged because the participants rushed things at the start and never knew how to cool down.

In the story that started this chapter, some students were tied together and played around, oblivious to the danger they were in. Look around you, see the canyon's edge, and notice that the rocks you're standing on are loose. You need to keep your balance. Don't lose yourself.

Hold off on the physical. Sex has power all its own. Intended as an expression of whole-person intimacy (and ultimately expressed within marriage), sexual activity can quickly defy those intentions and become the main event. Sex is a crooked politician, making wild promises just to get elected. Sex is a dark cloud hanging over the guilt-ridden. Sex is a weapon that frequently backfires. Sex is a treasure.

You meet someone you're attracted to. You begin the conquest. You do all the things that lead to a solid relationship, and things are going well. Then one fine night you get sexually involved with the person. And that changes everything. You have completed the conquest, and now you're not so interested.

Or maybe you're still interested, but your interest begins to focus on sex. Now the most important thing about that person is how he or she makes you feel sexually. The relationship is cheapened. You find it practically impossible to go on a date without ending up in bed.

You believe in saving sexual intercourse for marriage. But this new relationship is so hot, you go too far. Now you feel bound to this person. You've shared special intimacies. Maybe if you stay with this person, it will all be okay. The relationship crumbles around you, but you desperately hold on. You end up clinging to an unhealthy situation because you can't forgive yourself and start over.

Can you relate to any of these? These are just a few of the scenarios that occur when people rush into physical interaction.

Relationships quickly spin out of balance, especially when you have addictive tendencies in the first place. Obviously, there is a wide range of physical contact—from hand-holding to sexual intercourse. We're not going to give you a scorecard, just the strong caution: Hold back; be careful; go slowly; be strong. The health of this new relationship depends on it.

Set aside some time for yourself. I've already talked about limiting the frequency of your dates. This is the flip side of that strategy. One problem that keeps coming up in addictive relationships is that people lose themselves. They spend every waking hour (and some sleeping hours) with, planning to be with, thinking about, or dreaming about the object of their affection. They are consumed. They see themselves only as an adjunct to the other person, some sort of sidecar, the tick on the dog.

It is essential that you take time to nourish yourself, to get in touch with yourself, to remember who you are, apart from the other person. Establish this habit early in your relationship and it will strengthen you throughout. Set aside time to be alone: fifteen minutes a day, or two hours a week, or every Saturday morning or Sunday evening. This is time to be alone with yourself (or with God) and get grounded again.

Keep your friends. Don't let your lover decide who your friends will be. Sometimes this is done flagrantly, like when a jealous lover resents the time you spend with long-time pals. It can also be done subtly, as your lover gently discourages those other friendships or plans events so that you'll have to break dates with your friends. It can also be done by you, as you get so wrapped up in your new lover that you let old friendships slide.

Don't let this happen. First, let your partner know that your friendships are special to you and will continue to be (though you may have to assure your partner that there's no romantic threat).

Second, confront any subtle manipulation on the part of your lover and bring it out into the open: "I know you don't like Bill and Judy, but I've promised to have dinner with them this week. I'm not asking you to come, but I can't break that date to be with you. I'm sorry. It's not that they're more important to me than you are, but I do want to keep them as friends, and I do want to keep my promises."

Third, combat your own tendencies to neglect your friends. Work at restoring valuable friendships that may be slipping away.

Trust your friends' opinions. Your friends know you. They may know part of your romantic history. If you're entering a new romance, you probably have some blind spots. You need the outside opinions of those who know you best. They are not always right, but their opinions, combined with your own, are valuable. You may need to seek out their opinions. Sometimes friends will not venture to pry into your business. But if you ask them, they may provide some helpful cautions.

Communicate openly and honestly from the start. Misunderstandings that take root in the early days of a relationship can grow into conflicts that create great pain. "But I thought . . . ." "But you said . . . ." Years later you find yourself bound to a person you don't really know.

Early in a relationship, you want to assume that everything will be fine. You're looking through those rose-colored glasses and excusing all sorts of things. "Three hours late for a date? That's fine. I needed to catch up on my macramé." As a result, you don't establish the boundary lines that need to be set up. You can walk all over each other and never know it.

"I don't want him to think that I'm . . . a nag, a prude, a whiner, unfeeling, unsophisticated."

"I don't want her to think that I'm . . . a jerk, a prude, ignorant, poor, unconfident, unmasculine."

You know what this is like, don't you? We do the dance, presenting false images of ourselves and assuming the best about the other. (I heard a comic say, "I hate dates. You spend the whole night trying to pretend you're something you're not, hoping to get her to the point where she'll accept you for who you are.") Reality crashes in later, often with destructive results.

Be honest from the outset. Present yourself honestly and perceive the other person with the same honesty.

Talk through the conflicts, even if they seem minor. If you can learn to work through the minor differences, you've gone a long way toward establishing a healthy relationship.

Try saying something like, "You were three hours late and that really bothered me. It made me feel like you really don't care about me, and maybe that's true. I think you're worth another chance. If you're going to be late, you need to call. I deserve better treatment than what you just gave me." Boundaries, emotional disclosure, and self-esteem are all there. If you can say all that (and if it's accepted) there's hope for the relationship.

3. In a Relationship that's Becoming Addictive

So you're in this relationship. It has been maybe three or four months of dating and the two of you have grown together. Your dates and conversations are frequent and exclusive. Your worlds are beginning to revolve around each other. But something is vaguely bothersome.

Then you read a book like this one, and you begin to recognize some of the danger zones. "Yeah, that's us," you say. "I am losing myself. This relationship is built on need."

What do you do?

Or maybe you've been in the relationship for a long time, but it has been changing recently. A crisis has changed you or the other person. Perhaps an addiction of some kind has surfaced. Whatever, you begin to notice these addictive symptoms in your relationship.

What do you do?

You're on the slope, but not far down it. The problems have begun to appear, but they're not deep-seated. This is the region of "no easy answers." Can the relationship be saved? Maybe. Maybe not.

Just like Annie and Barry, you've lost your footing, but you may be able to climb back out together. They helped each other, practically leapfrogging their way back up the slope. If you're determined to have a healthy relationship, sometimes you can pull each other back to a safer spot.

Evaluate the relationship—and the danger. Does this have the potential of being a healthy relationship? Is the relationship so good that it has to be saved? This is a Catch-22 question, along the lines of "Are you a compulsive liar?" If you're addicted, naturally you'll say, "Yes, yes, this relationship is the best thing that's ever happened to me!"—even if it isn't. You may need to rely on outside opinions from friends and family.

Does the other person strengthen you? This is a key approach. The question is not: Does the other person make up for your mistakes? Or: Does the other person make you feel better? Or even: Does the other person meet your needs? But: Does the other person make you stronger? It's the difference between being an *enabler* (in the modern recovery lingo) and an *empowerer*. An *enabler* merely allows you to continue functioning in a dependent way. An *empowerer* helps you toward independence and interdependence.

If this person were taken away from you, naturally it would hurt you. But would you be at a total loss? Or would you be able to function on your own?

Your relationship may have some addictive elements, but if there is true empowering going on, there is hope for it.

How important is the relationship to you? When you look at this romance in the clear light of day, is it something you want to sink your life into? Is it something you want to put a lot of work into? Or is it filling a temporary need in your life? If the relationship is not worth all that much to you, get out if you sense that it's becoming addictive. Get out while you still can—it will only get harder as time goes on.

What practical considerations apply? How interwoven is your life with your lover's life? Can you get out now? In the case of marriage, there's a whole different set of rules. You have to make that work, if you can. But perhaps you're dating a coworker or a neighbor. The proximity of these people can create extra ropes to bind you into the relationship trap, much like the kids in the story—at the edge of the cliff and all tangled up with each other. You need to be aware of these practical constraints, and do what you can to remain unsnared.

If you decide to end the relationship, move on to situations 4 and 5. Since the addiction is just beginning, it won't be as serious as the cases of those who are well-entrenched, but the same principles apply.

If you think it's best to stay in the relationship, but to try to make it less addictive, read on.

Agree together to change things. It takes two to tangle—and to untangle. Talk together about the addictive nature of your relationship. Discuss how you want things to be between you, and what a healthy love in which both partners are honored would look like. If your partner does not agree to work through this with you, your chances of restoration are slim to none.

Consider taking a vacation from each other. Yes, such vacations are often just the prelude to a breakup. But they can also provide valuable rebuilding time for the individuals involved. In addictive relationships, people need to restore and protect their sense of self, apart from the other person. Set aside a couple of weeks to a month when you will not see each other or have any contact (except maybe by phone). You'll probably learn a lot about yourself—and the relationship. You may find that you're better off without the other person, or you may come back together that much stronger.

Stop the physical relationship. At least for a time, set stark new boundaries on your physical interaction. Say, "For the next month, let's try just kissing goodnight at the door."

This is not just prudery, but discipline. Consider it an experiment or a corrective procedure. It will be terribly frustrating if you are used to sexual intimacy. But it should be a helpful rebalancing of your relationship.

Sex throws things out of balance. The "intimacy" it provides is shallow, often need-oriented and one-sided. When sexual intimacy is not supported by whole-person commitment, it can contribute to an addiction.

Calling a moratorium, even a temporary one, on the sexual interaction can help the other aspects of the relationship to catch up. You can discover whole new sides to this other person. On the other hand, if you are unable to be non-physical for even a month, how healthy is that relationship?

Build or rebuild outside friendships. As I said before, addictive relationships can destroy other friendships. You zero in on your lover and no one else matters. You can put the brakes on this by making a point to maintain your friendships or make new friends. You may have already alienated some old friends. Try to win them back by asking for forgiveness, expressing how much you need them at this time (and promising to be there for them).

Create some personal time or personal projects for yourself. To keep from losing yourself in the relationship, set aside time to be by yourself. Or consider taking on a new, self-building project. Join a theater group or take piano lessons or tutor inner-city kids. It's important that you do this on your own, and not involve your partner. If your partner resists your attempts at self-building, he or she is exerting too much control over you. You need to grow so that you can be a fuller person, as well as a whole partner in the relationship. If your partner can't accept that, you need to jump ship.

Keep a journal. As I said in the last chapter, journal-keeping has numerous benefits. It gets you in touch with your own feelings, and it serves as a record that you can consult later when your memory plays tricks on you.

4. When You're in a Relationship that Is Deeply Addictive

You're farther down the slope. You are solidly in the relationship and solidly addicted to it. Your life is about this other person.

You have forgotten who you are; you think of yourself only in relation to your partner. What can you do to save this relationship, to make it healthy again?

Nothing.

Like the kids in the story that began this chapter, you must cut the rope and run out the other side. You can't climb back up the slope. The relationship is doomed.

What do you need to do for yourself? Get out of the relationship as quickly and cleanly as you can. In our story, it was Frank who had the right idea, cutting loose from Sarah and running for help.

It won't be easy. It's like the junkie quitting drugs cold turkey. You have to decide to do it and then do what you've decided. There will be all sorts of forces compelling you to stay in the relationship, not least of which is your partner. But you must be strong and get out. *You will not find personal healing until you do*. Now how do you accomplish this huge deed? I have no magic words, just a few ideas.

Decide to do it. It almost goes without saying, but you need to make up your mind that you're going to break off the relationship. And not because this book tells you to or because anyone else decides it's best. You need to decide for yourself. (You may want to go back and review chapter 9 and apply those principles.)

Know why you're doing it. What reasons do you have? How is the relationship unhealthy for you? Make a list, so you're clear about this. This list is not for anyone else, just for you. You don't need to convince your partner that these reasons are valid, you just need to convince yourself. If you waver, go back to the list. (Here's where previous journaling will help.)

Build your own personal strength and self-esteem. This might actually be step one. If you know you need to break up, but you don't think you can, go on a self-building campaign. Tell yourself good things about yourself. Hang around people who like you and show it. Addictive relationships tend to knock down your self-esteem, and that saps your strength. Building yourself up will put you in position to make this difficult break.

Decide when, where and how you will make the break. Don't make vague promises to yourself. Be specific. "Monday at lunch, we'll talk and I'll do it."

Rely on friends for moral support and accountability. Let them remind you why you're breaking up. Let them encourage you. Don't be afraid to ask them for encouragement. Let a few close friends know when you are planning to break up and ask them to hold you accountable. You have to go through with it then, or you'll be letting them down.

Don't be afraid to cause a scene or look foolish or act mean or cause pain. No one wants to be the bad guy. Not one of us wants to hurt someone we care about. But this is something that has to be done, and there's no nice way to do it. Your partner may cry or yell or whimper or hit you or hate you. Be prepared for all of that and steel yourself. There is probably no gentle way to do this.

Think of yourself as a parent taking a child to the doctor for a much-needed shot. It will hurt, and the parent hates the child's pain as much as the child does. But it must be done. No matter how much the child whimpers and whines, the loving parent will go through with it. It is far better for the child in the long run to endure the pain and accept the shot's healing power. You are administering a necessary shot that will be best for both you and your partner.

You may want to choose a public location for the breakup conversation to prevent your partner from attacking or seducing you. (Lovers can fight back in either way.) You may want to leave yourself an out, such as paying for lunch beforehand so you can leave if things get too heated. Don't respond to a partner's threat to cause a scene in a public place. It may be embarrassing for the moment, but it's not worth undoing the good thing you've done.

Don't give it "one more chance." You've made your decision. Stick with it. There have probably been numerous "one more chances" before. Don't buy it. This may seem unreasonable on your part, but don't worry about being unreasonable. You need to hold to your decision. Be aware of new evidence your partner may bring in to try to keep you. By this I mean something new, maybe even surprising, that your partner has never done or said before—making promises, proposing marriage. When your partner realizes you're serious, he or she will do all sorts of things to change your mind, to get you thinking, "Maybe it will be different this time."

It won't be different. Go through with the breakup. If those promises, that "new evidence," has any validity, you'll have to examine it later, much later, when you're free from the addictive trap. Right now, don't let anything diminish your resolve.

After the breakup, avoid the other person. You can't be friends. Staying friends seems like the nice thing to do, but it is far too risky. You will likely be pulled right back into the addiction. The "just friends" line is something you may want to say during the breakup conversation to ease the pain, but it doesn't work in real life.

This may require bold action. If you're working with the person, you may need to request a transfer or even change jobs. (I realize that's easier said than done, but your emotional health might require it.) If you live near the person, you may need to move, or at least change your normal route so you don't run into the person. (More about avoiding the person in situation 6.)

5. If You Feel It's Impossible to Go Cold Turkey

When you're in the very bottom of the pit, you feel as if you can't make it. You're tempted to give up, because after all, "Isn't a bad relationship better than no relationship at all?" No, it's not. But I know it can be hard to convince yourself of that.

Try anyway. It's a difficult process, but I really don't see any other way of attaining the healing you need. Grit your teeth and do it. *There's no easy way out of an addiction.* I can't make this any plainer: Just as you can't gradually stop taking drugs or take a drink only once a month to wean yourself off of alcoholism, you can't stop an addictive relationship without a clean break.

See a professional counselor. We're not always miracle workers, but we can help you through some difficult decisions. Through our training and experience, we have some insights to share about the nature of relationships: what's healthy, what's not, and what might be some of your roadblocks in making a clean break.

Find a counselor you're comfortable with. Ask friends for their recommendations, but you should also ask your pastor or doctor for their referrals. If you feel uncomfortable with a counselor you visit, say so. The counselor may learn to accommodate your needs in a better way or may refer you to someone who matches your needs better. Remember, it is always up to you to choose a counselor, go to your sessions, communicate what you need, and ultimately to change. You can see how well a particular counselor helps you, gain some insights, and then try a different counselor if you like. It's up to you, but you should seek some kind of help.

Put up strong boundaries and live by them. Let me say it again: *This is second-best; the best recovery is still cold turkey.* But if you absolutely cannot make a clean break, at least try to put the brakes on the addiction by setting limits.

Consider limiting your physical relationship, your amount of time together, the money that you spend on the other person (or that is spent on you), or the areas in which you rely on the other person. If you have determined that you or your partner is overly dependent in some area, make up your mind to change that area. This is a matter of treating the symptoms, but it may help.

Avoid drugs and alcohol. This is a dangerous time for you. If you're addicted to a relationship, you are very susceptible to other addictions as well. I've known many who have let their dissatisfaction with their relationships and their inability to break free drive them to drink or use drugs. These, of course, just make things worse. These "cross-addictions" are very common among those with addictive personalities.

If you are experiencing physical or sexual abuse, get out and get help. There are cases of relationship severe addiction where husbands regularly beat their wives and the wives feel powerless to change things. If this is your situation, you're not doing anyone a favor by keeping silent. Your husband needs help and so do you. If there are children involved, they definitely need help, too.

Many communities have special hotlines for battered women. (Often these are listed in the "blue pages" of your phone book.) Call one of these, or call the police (especially in violent or dangerous situations). Consult with your pastor and/or other church leaders. Ask your doctor to recommend an agency that might help. Do not keep the secret any longer.

6. Once You're Out of an Addictive Relationship

Let's say you've done it. You've recognized your addiction and taken the necessary steps to get out of the problem relationship. Great! But you're not out of the woods yet. Relapse is common, unless you remain vigilant. Continue to gather the strength you need to stay free from your ex-partner and from new addictive relationships.

Stay away from your ex-partner. As I said before, it's tempting to be "just friends." But it doesn't work. You see, in most cases it's not just an addiction to a romance with that person, it's an addiction to a friendship, too. You've learned to rely on that person for all sorts of things, and after the breakup you will miss that person terribly. You might assume that if the romance is ended, the danger of addiction is gone, and so the friendship can continue. The addiction can go on in the friendship, and that may lead you back into a romance.

One young couple I counseled had just broken off an unhealthy romance but continued (against my advice) to see each other as friends. Jenny had initiated the breakup, which hurt Will deeply, but she felt sorry for him and still invited him for dinner each week. On one of these occasions, Jenny (perhaps missing their old times together) came on to Will sexually, and they ended up in bed together. Like Scott in chapter 6, he too left even more confused and distraught than before.

They have since agreed that it's best to stay away from each other entirely. It is just too difficult to maintain proper boundaries when you continue to see your former addiction.

Other recovering addicts know this well. Recovering alcoholics do not hang around bars. Recovering drug abusers avoid their old suppliers. Similarly, recovering relationship addicts need to avoid the people they've been addicted to.

Don't rationalize—just stay away! I've known people who planned to "accidentally" bump into their old lovers. They missed the relationship and just wanted to see the person, but wanted to assure themselves they were still going cold turkey. So they'd drive by the person's house or office, and ultimately arrange to meet.

Will was one of these people. He had left a bunch of stuff at Jenny's place. Each week or so he had an excuse to go back and fetch something—and to see her, of course. "Just make one trip," I told him. "Take a big box and get all your stuff out of there." But he felt he needed that excuse.

He kept in touch with Jenny's friends. If they were going out somewhere together, he would just "happen" to show up there. The truth was, he was continuing to feed his addiction. Part of him agreed that a clean break was necessary, but another part kept lying to himself, finding flimsy excuses to see Jenny again.

"What does it hurt?" Will asked me. "I just saw Jenny briefly. Nothing happened. I just needed to see her. What's the problem with that?"

"You're addicted," I replied. "Try saying the same thing, but substituting the word 'cocaine' for Jenny."

He tried it. "What does it hurt?" he said tentatively. "I just . . . did a little cocaine. I just needed it. What's the problem with that?"

We looked at each other and he knew what the problem was. It is foolish and dangerous to continue seeing the object of your addiction. Stay away, and don't kid yourself.

Admit your ongoing addictive tendency. One of the helpful insights from twelve-step groups is that you continue to be an addict even when you've kicked the habit. You're in recovery, but you're still susceptible. The alcoholic stands at the AA meeting and says, "My name is Bob and I am an alcoholic. It's been twenty years since my last drink." Day after day he recognizes his weakness and fights it. Those days have stretched into twenty sober years.

Even when you leave an addictive relationship, you carry a susceptibility to relational addictions. You must be careful about future relationships. Perhaps even twenty years from now.

Reject the rebound. When a well-meaning friend says, "You need a new love in your life," say, "No, I don't." Rebound relationships can sneak up on you. There is great emotional and social pressure to plunge in again. Don't do it.

"This new guy will make you forget all about Richard." "One date with Sheila and your feelings for Marie are history."

Don't buy it. It's like taking heroin to forget about cocaine, like swilling gin to kick your vodka habit. It doesn't help.

Take time to heal. People want instant cures for long-term problems. I've known people who took twenty years to develop a smoking habit, yet they want to be cured in twenty minutes. Sure, God works miracles. But the miracle of healing usually takes place over a period of time. Relationship addiction is no different.

I work with people recovering from divorce. They're often amazed when I recommend that they wait at least two years before staring a new romance. Two years! You'd think I just asked them to enter a monastery. But the truth is that most people aren't ready to re-enter the dating world for about two years, longer for some. If your addictive relationship was long-term, that might be a good bench mark for you. Use those two years to recover, to build your self-image, to build healthy friendships, but not to find a new lover.

If your relationship was of shorter duration or less serious, a shorter recovery period may suffice—perhaps six months to a year. Think of it this way: As long as it took you to get into that relationship, it will probably take you at least that long to get out.

Watch out for other forms of addiction. Drugs, alcohol, gambling, pornography, food, and other addictive substances may try to sneak up on you.

Develop a positive program for yourself. So far, I've been saying, "Don't." Here's one more caution: Don't dwell on the negative. Get a plan to put yourself back together. Go to the gym on a regular basis. Read the books you've always wanted to read. Start a Thursday night video party to catch up on the classics. Go to church and volunteer to help with the refreshments. Get out your old guitar and try to remember the chords.

This is a time to rebuild yourself. Whatever your action plan is, tackle it with all your might.

Rebuild friendships and social supports. You need close friends more than ever. If you have alienated old friends, restore those friendships.

Get involved with groups, too. Enlarge your circle of acquaintances. Singles groups become a great deal of fun when you stop trying to hook someone of the opposite sex. But don't limit yourself to singles groups. There are service organizations, softball teams, study groups, bowling leagues, community theaters, political campaigns, and neighborhood groups to join.

Develop safe friendships with the opposite sex. You may not be ready immediately. You may go through a "Men Are Jerks" or "Women Are Stupid" phase. But maybe six months after your breakup, you should make it a point to get to know someone of the opposite sex in a safe, non-romantic way. This can begin to restore your image of the other gender. Amazingly, some men can really listen to you. Some women can be brilliant.

There are men who can talk about things other than sports. There are women who can be honest with you. That may be hard to believe in the wake of your breakup, but you need to learn that eventually.

Get in touch with your purpose in life. Think about why you're here. On the earth. Living life.

You don't need to come up with a well-defined "purpose statement," unless you enjoy doing that sort of thing. Expect that there will always be some mysteries concerning our existence here, even though we may have a general idea of what we're about. But think about your purpose.

Then, when you've thought about it, do something in keeping with it.

Do a good deed for a neighbor. Go grocery shopping for the elderly woman next door. Buy a Big Mac for the homeless person who hassles you on the street. Encourage a troubled family member. Teach an inner-city kid to count to ten. Go to church and sing God's praises for all you're worth. Spend time praying for the needs of those around you.

Acts like these can get you in the right groove again. They can remind you of how valuable you are. They can anchor you and keep you from sliding down Addiction Canyon again.

CHAPTER ELEVEN

Case Study: Laurie

ℒ

LAURIE IS AN EXCEPTION. MOST ADDICTIONS HAVE DEEP-SEATED CAUSES, but Laurie's came on suddenly. Most carry ongoing dangers, but Laurie's struggle now seems to be finished. We might call it a catastrophic addiction. Her life was not an addiction waiting to happen, but it happened anyway. Her case serves to remind us that anyone can succumb to a relationship addiction, and anyone can recover from it.

She sits in my office now, not as a counselee, but as a former client. She's telling me her story again, for this book, hoping it helps others. She is the picture of a confident, healthy, whole person. The events she describes are five years in the past. Only within the last year, she says, has she finally put it behind her.

Breaking the Rules

In her mid-forties, Laurie has been married and divorced twice. Her first husband was a philanderer. She remains friends with her second—that marriage "just didn't work out." Her addiction began shortly after her second divorce.

She's quick to say that she was not "on the rebound." Her second marriage had been crumbling for a while. She is well aware of the slippery slope of divorce recovery, and she says she was through that. She was not a wreck at the time. No, she seemed healthy and well-adjusted as she re-entered single life. "I was not emotionally vulnerable," she says now, looking back. "I thought I knew what I was doing. Well, I was wrong."

Forced to support herself, Laurie got a job in a financial consulting office, where she learned the ropes quickly. There she met Alan.

Alan was a hunk. He had a winning personality and a sense of humor that made him a good businessman—and popular with women. He was no flashy flirt, either. He seemed sincerely interested in people, especially in Laurie. When he started to come on to her, she couldn't believe her good fortune.

"I broke my own rule," she says. "'Never get involved with anyone you work with. I should have known better."

But he was overwhelming, saying the right things, doing the right things. Their romance blossomed. They dated for about six months and then they moved in together.

"It was good for a few months after that," Laurie says. "But then he started to withdraw. He would do things on his own without telling me. He wouldn't include me in things." Alan had an opportunity to buy a house at a good price. That was his excuse to move out, though they continued their relationship.

"He was great at mixed messages. When he was with me, he said all the things I wanted to hear. He was a master at that. But there were a lot of things he just wasn't telling me."

Like, he was seeing someone else.

Laurie found that out a month after he moved out. She was furious. "He didn't deny it, he didn't defend himself, he didn't do anything. That's the way he is." Laurie's voice is calm as she describes those events, but her tone bears the scars of a lot of hurt. She must have been fuming at the time.

She had run headlong into that maddening male passivity.

She had assumed his unmixed devotion to her. But as he saw it, he had made no promises, so he was free to date her and anyone else who came along.

But she wasn't. Her heart was wrapped around his life. She was addicted.

Alan continued to "waltz in and out" of Laurie's life for the next year. She saw him daily at work, and they would date occasionally. Their times together were great; he was charming as usual. But there was always the specter of those "other women" he was seeing. She wanted him all to herself. Whenever they did go out, she'd feel great for a few days, and then fall apart. She had the sense that she was a second choice for him, and yet she longed to be with him. Her self-esteem, normally quite healthy, was sliding.

Then he stopped asking Laurie out. There was one "other woman" he wanted to focus his attention on. He would not be dating Laurie anymore.

She was destroyed. Though, in retrospect, this was probably the best thing for her, at the time she was devastated.

"I couldn't sleep. I developed a cough that I couldn't get rid of. My hair started falling out. I had a horrible feeling in my chest and in my stomach. I was frequently under medication and very suicidal. I used to pray, 'Lord, if you love me, put me out of my misery.' I wanted to die more than anything because I just didn't want to face the pain. I remember screaming at the Lord, punching the walls, hitting my head against the walls, scratching my face, doing things that seem totally bizarre to me now."

That was when she came to see me for counseling.

The Road to Recovery

What do you say to such a person? Basically, you try to empower her to pick herself up and start over, to make the hard decisions she needs to make. You try to help her get a realistic perspective on her life and relationships. You assure her of her personal worth. You put her in contact with other people facing similar struggles (which is why I asked her to join our circle).

Laurie's pain was intensified by the fact that she worked closely with Alan. He also lived down the street from her. And he wanted to stay friends. It was all smiles in the office, though inside Laurie was burning up. My normal "cold turkey" advice would be to get a new job and move away. But Laurie wouldn't do this, and I don't blame her. She had a good job. She had risen in the company and now commanded an impressive salary. Through all this crisis, her performance at work had not suffered. She prided herself on that. She felt like a "slimeball" in the rest of her life, but she still acted with confidence at work. It was a bit of certainty she didn't want to give up.

So the next solution was to close the door to any future romantic involvement with Alan. He had waltzed through her heart with abandon for the last year. Even though he had rejected her now, he was not burning any bridges. She felt the distinct possibility that he might come back to her if his current relationship didn't work out. She secretly hoped for this.

But that would just put her back on the roller coaster, back into the addiction. She needed to break from him, to slam the door. Otherwise she would never be free.

One winter day, Laurie went through her home and picked up every item that belonged to Alan. She put it all in a big box. It was a purging of the last two years of her life. Every remnant of his life with her was piled together in that box. He did not belong in her home anymore. She drove down the street to his house and deposited the box at his door.

That was a major act in her recovery. But one thing remained. Alan still had a key to her place. She needed to get it back. It seems like such a trifle. He certainly wouldn't use it since he had moved on to another relationship. There was no danger involved. But that key was a symbol of something much greater—his right to reenter her life romantically. I urged her to get the key back. She assured me she would.

But she forgot. And she forgot again. And she forgot again. She saw him frequently at work but was not asking for the key. "I think part of me wanted him to have that key," Laurie says now.

About a month after she left the box at his door, Laurie asked Alan for her key. It was a few more weeks before she got it. A chapter of her life had finally ended. And a new one began: recovery, the healing of her heart. It's not easy when the scab is regularly ripped open at work. "Being in an addictive relationship is the worst thing I can think of," she says. "It's worse than being on drugs, I think. It's awful to have to see a person every day, someone you really care about and really love, and to know that that person is going on with his life without you. I don't know how I got through it. I had a lot of people there who loved me and supported me, and I drew strength from my relationship with God."

Laurie began to keep a journal, which was a helpful outlet for her feelings. She also found our group sessions helpful. She appreciated and needed the encouragement of others who were in the same boat. But it has been, quite literally, a day-to-day struggle. Alan continued his winsome ways at work. And Laurie never knew when she would see him with another woman as she drove by his house.

It was about four years ago that Laurie finally got her key back. Her healing has been slow but sure.

At one point, Alan was away from the office for a few months, and that was good. But he came back.

Then he was having problems with his steady girlfriend, and that was bad. "He had the nerve to ask me out again. It was all I could do to say no." This was what she had dreamed of earlier, her second chance with the man she loved. But she had made some hard choices by that time. The door was closed. "It hadn't stopped hurting; I just made up my mind that this relationship could not be. Maybe at that point it was my pride. I just couldn't let him yank me around like that any more."

Now she seems strong again, brimming with self-esteem. She still sees Alan at the office. "I am able to work with him and it doesn't hurt," she tells me as she sits in my office. "I even get annoyed at him sometimes." She says she recently worked closely on a project with him and felt no emotional pain. It's over.

Hindsight

"If I had gone cold turkey, not seeing him at all," she says, "it would have been painful, but the healing would not have lasted this long. With cold turkey, you have the blessing of not having to see the person or talk to him or know what's going on in his life. I didn't have that option. I was exposed to it every day."

She seems to have gained confidence through the ordeal. And she is in no hurry for a new romance. "I have no intention of ever having any repeats," she laughs.

"I have some pretty close relationships with some men," she goes on, "but they're not romantic. I haven't met anybody I desire to have a romantic relationship with. I think my expectations are much higher. I'm at the point where I see dysfunctional behavior or some quirk in a man and I just don't pursue it."

Laurie speaks about the boundaries she has discovered. She won't lose herself in a man again. "I'm okay on my own. I wouldn't mind being in a relationship, but I don't need it. I'm who I am and I'm happy with who I am now. I just got to the point where I said, 'Okay, you have to be a healthy person and be happy with Laurie, whether there's someone else in your life or not.'"

She says she can sympathize with people who are in similar situations. She'd like to use her experience to help people who are hurting. "Whether through divorce or the loss of a child, I think I have a lot to give. I've walked on the hot coals for a long time and I've learned an awful lot and I want to give it back."

What advice does she give to those who are where she was, wrestling with a relationship addiction? "I would tell them to quit, to get as far away from the situation as they possibly could. If that's not an option, I'd urge them to talk to a professional counselor. They need a group of friends who can encourage them, friends who are honest enough to tell you the truth whether you want to hear it or not. Pray. Put your life in God's hands. It may take God a long time to answer—but He does answer. And be strong. Realize that you have a lot of value as a human being and you have a lot of value in the eyes of God. Look for ways that this can make you stronger."

Evaluation

Laurie has no serious addiction in her family history. But she does seem to have some compulsion to be in a romantic relationship. Her recent troubles have scared her off of such relationships for a while, but this is the longest she has ever gone "without a man."

Her difficulty with Alan could be due to her idealization of him. She looked up to him professionally and admired him physically. Her need for a relationship allowed her to ignore the mistreatment she received from Alan—things she never would have tolerated from either of her husbands. This confirms a point we've been seeing: Addictive relationships are irrational. They can't always be explained and rarely make sense. By all appearances, Laurie should have been able to stand up to Alan and avoid these complications. Why didn't she? That's one of those irrationalities.

But there is hope. Laurie has come through this struggle to become a stronger person. That can happen to many others in similar situations. With professional help, the support of close friends, and an awareness of their personal value and purpose in life, wounded people can break the addictive grip and come back to health and freedom.

CHAPTER TWELVE

Best Friends

🙠

T HE COACH YELLS FROM THE FIRST-BASE LINE: "SEE YOURSELF HITTING
the ball, Joey! See that level swing! See yourself making
contact!"

The coach had obviously coached Joey before; he was
reminding him to keep his right elbow up, to keep his eye on the
ball. Then he said, "See yourself hitting the ball." As Joey con-
centrated, I was reminded of the importance of maintaining a
vision of our relational goals as well, the benefits of focusing on
healthy love.

There's a sports theory called *psychocybernetics*.

The idea is that your body conforms to what you see—or
what you imagine yourself seeing. Even if you don't know how
to move all those muscles in just the right way, your body knows,
and it will perform correctly if you give it a proper image.

I don't know if that's a valid sports strategy or not. (In Joey's
case, he must have seen himself hitting a pop-up to the short-
stop.) But it is a valid relationship strategy.

Many people have faulty relationships because they don't
know any better. They've never seen a good relationship in action.
We have seen this in our case studies: people are repeating the

dysfunctions of their birth families. Girls crave attention from their fathers and grow up to crave attention from their husbands. Men are self-centered rogues and women are stupid servants—that's all some people have ever known.

As you strive to develop and maintain healthy relationships, you need to have good images in front of you. Find couples with solid marriages and see how they do it. Stop watching TV shows about dysfunctional families and try to find shows that show mutually committed relationships (good luck!). Read the rest of this chapter to see what relational health really looks like. And then see yourself in a healthy relationship.

Good relationships are characterized by three things: best friendship, balance, and boundaries. We'll talk first about being your partner's best friend.

Best Friendship

Healthy romances are also good friendships. Sad to say, this isn't true of all romances. You probably know people who say about their partners:

"He really turns me on, but I don't feel that I know him at all."

"She's a lot of fun to go out with, but I don't really trust her."

"I love the way she looks, but I don't understand her. When we talk, it's like we're in different worlds."

"I feel so afraid when I'm with him. I can't really be myself."

Romantic attraction is a capricious thing; it flies on whims and impulse. The ancients depicted the god Cupid firing his arrows, often at random. If you fall in love with someone who's good for you, you're lucky. When relationships are only built on feelings, they're unsteady. They can crash with the first strong wind.

But how do friendships happen? Usually, you find someone among your acquaintances who shares your interests. Perhaps you find you think alike in certain areas or that your personalities are complementary. Consciously or subconsciously, you decide to spend more time together, to share more deeply of yourself, to listen to and care for the other person. The friendship grows on such sharing. Friendships grown and nurtured through time can weather all sorts of difficulties.

Can you have both romance and friendship? Yes. Many couples have started out in torrid romances, only to have those feelings fade. But, in the place of those romantic feelings, they find that a new friendship has been forged. This doesn't happen automatically. It requires communication, trust, and committed love.

Communication

Best friends can talk about anything and everything. They are interested in each other's lives and feel free to express their own feelings. Each one understands how the other's mind works. They don't always agree, but when they do, they understand their disagreements. They don't get hung up on petty quarrels because they know where the other person is coming from.

Volumes have been written on the art of communication. If you're having problems communicating with your partner, consult one of those. We don't have room here for a full treatment, but let me suggest some areas that might require attention.

First, at least half of the communication process is listening. That goes without saying, right? But I'm amazed at how many couples get in trouble because they stop listening to each other. Sometimes we assume we know what the other person is saying, so we tune out. Sometimes we're so concerned about making our own point that we never focus on what the other person is saying. Sometimes we read negative motives into the other person's statements, and we react defensively to imaginary attacks.

"Stop, look, and listen" might be a catch-phrase for healthy relationships. Good listeners are not afraid to say, "Would you repeat that?" or "What do you mean by that?" in an effort to clarify what they heard. They may repeat the statement in a different way to make sure they've got it right. "Do you really mean to say that you think baseball is the best game ever invented?"

Second, good communicators know how to make "I statements." An "I statement" says how I feel, without attributing motives or feelings to anyone else. If I say, "You're so selfish!", I'm setting up for a fight. But if I turn that into an "I statement"— "When I see you act that way, it makes me feel like you don't care about me"—then we can deal peacefully with the problem. My partner is not on the defensive. On the contrary, I've made myself vulnerable.

It's possible that my partner could respond, "Well, you're imagining things, as usual" or "You're just too sensitive." But I'm banking on the fact that my partner is as interested as I am in resolving our conflicts. I'm giving her the benefit of the doubt. I'm implying, "I believe you do care about me, even though I'm not reading that in your behavior. So either I'm reading you wrong or you're not expressing your love for me. Let's work on this together." (If your partner consistently responds to your "I statements" with further attacks on you, then perhaps these assumptions are not true. In that case, your problem is greater than just poor communication.)

Practicing communication this way brings the discussion back to the basics of where *I* am, what *I* feel. It also allows for the possibility that I may be wrong in my interpretation of the other person's actions or words. It's an important tactic in any couple's attempt to maintain good communication.

Some people say, "We don't need to talk. We know each other so well, we read each other's minds." Maybe so, but that sounds to me like unrealistic romanticizing. It can be terribly frustrating when you think you're reading your partner's mind, but your translation is dead wrong. And it can be threatening to have your mind read. (I saw a cartoon once in which a character said, "I know you think you know what I thought when I said that, but I really thought something else, I think.") For a healthy relationship, you need to keep talking—if only to verify and calibrate your mind-reading skills.

In his witty drama *Our Town*, Thornton Wilder shows a middle-aged couple having breakfast on their son's wedding day. Dr. Gibbs says, "Julia, do you know one of the things I was scared of when I married you? . . . I was afraid we wouldn't have material for conversation more'n'd last us a few weeks."

They laugh together, and he adds, "Well, you and I have been conversing for twenty years now without any noticeable barren spells."

"Well," his wife answers, "good weather, bad weather—'tain't very choice, but I always find something to say."

Granted, some people are gifted conversationalists; others aren't. But communication is essential to the health of a relationship. It doesn't have to be smooth or witty or entertaining or deeply sensitive. But it does need to happen.

Trust and Honor

Friendship involves trust. A friend can share something deeply personal, perhaps something shocking, and trust that the other person will remain loyal. Healthy relationships are based on that kind of trust and loyalty.

I'm not saying that you put your mind on hold. I'm not saying that you ignore dangerous situations. If your friend says he's beginning to use drugs, you'll express your friendship by helping him stop. You don't need to approve of bad behavior. But there's a commitment to the *person*. While you may need to express concern over some behaviors or attitudes, a true friend also expresses acceptance of the person.

When trust exists between two partners in a romantic relationship, there's openness and honesty. If I can trust you with my secrets, I'll begin to open up to you and build intimacy. I won't be afraid that I'm not good enough for you. Instead, I'll share myself with you.

In one of our case studies Sally spoke of "not being herself" with one man she dated. She thought he was out of her league and she was always trying to live up to his standards.

There was no openness there. She didn't trust him with her true self, and thus she maintained an off-balance relationship.

Obviously, trust is a two-way street. You need to earn my trust, and I yours. (In Sally's case, her lawyer friend obviously hadn't earned her trust; she would have been foolish to trust him with any more of herself. But that's a symptom of a bad relationship.) We earn trust by being loyal, by accepting, by (here's a key word) *honoring* the other person.

Do you know couples who honor each other? You'll be talking to one partner, and he'll say, "You really ought to ask my wife about that; she's brilliant on that subject." Or she'll say, "My husband did the sweetest thing, let me tell you about it." Yes, that can go to extremes when people dote on each other, but how refreshing it is to see that upbuilding going on! And just imagine what goes on at home. One says: "Honey, I think you ought to go ahead and take that art class. I think you'd be good at that." The other: "I'm sorry you didn't get that promotion. You earned it."

You may have met couples who take every opportunity to tear each other down. She'll give you play-by-play of his latest business failure. He'll make snide comments about her clothes, her looks, her age. They make everybody feel uncomfortable. You don't even want to imagine their home life.

Self-esteem is fragile. We bruise easily. Every time we open our mouths, we make ourselves vulnerable. Every time we say something about what's inside of us, we hand someone a knife. No wonder there are so many fearful people out there. They may be in relationships, but they feel lonely because they·have never felt secure enough to share what's inside of them.

It's easy to tear others down, but it's rewarding to build them up. In healthy relationships, partners honor each other, and by doing so they coax the other out of his or her shell. They inspire trust, openness and honesty.

It doesn't come all at once. Trust builds slowly. But at least a spark of it exists in every healthy relationship.

Self-giving Love

My colleague Tom Jones, in his book *The Single Again Handbook*, tells of a man who was leaving his wife Margie for a new love, Beth. The man spoke of how he hadn't "felt anything" with Margie for two years, and how Beth was giving him great new feelings.

Jones challenged him: Would these great new feelings last?

The man didn't know. He figured, "You just have to go with the feelings you have at the present."

"What is this feeling you have for Beth?" Jones asked. "Is it love?"

"If this isn't love," the man responded, "then I don't know what love is."

Jones concluded that the man was right—he didn't know what love was. Within two years he divorced Beth and asked Margie to take him back.

The story could be repeated in millions of homes. It's symptomatic of a deep problem: *We don't know what love is.*

A lot of what we call love is just shared enjoyment. "I love you because you make me feel so good, but when that feeling stops, babe—when you get wrinkles or I get bored—I'm out of here."

A lot of "love" is actually bargaining. I may be doing something nice for my partner, but I have an ulterior motive. I want some kind of payback. I'll do the dishes for her so that she won't put up a fuss when I have to go to a meeting tonight. In long-term relationships, you learn what you have to do to get along. Now there's nothing wrong with getting along—it's just not the *essence* of love.

Various writers have looked for love in ancient Greek words. The Greeks had four different words for different aspects of what we call love. The first, *storge*, is simple enjoyment. I "love" broccoli, cats, or baseball. The second, *eros*, is sexual love, the physical desire we feel for someone attractive. The third is *philia* or friendship. We tend to like those who are like us. In a way, in casual friendships we are loving ourselves, bonding with those who are going in the same direction as we are. You may have had friendships in your own life that you thought were pretty sturdy, but they crumbled when someone moved away or changed or got irked over some trivial matter. *Philia* is good, but it's not the ultimate kind of love.

Agape (uh-GAH-pay) is the final Greek word for love. This is the word the early Christians grabbed to describe the way God loves humans and how He wants us to love each other. It is love with no selfishness, no bargaining, no expectation of reward. It is a giving love. That's the kind of "best friendship" that healthy relationships have—not a casual shared-interest acquaintance, but a self-giving love.

Some people call this unconditional love. That's a great concept, but I think it invites misunderstanding. It's true that partners should love each other in a giving way, not just to receive something in return. The misunderstanding arises when we confuse unconditional love with codependency. True love looks out for the best interests of the other person. Thus it can be "tough love"—it calls the other person to accountability. Love does not enable people to carry on self-destructive behaviors. It empowers them to change, inspires them to step forward, and is patient as they stumble along.

One person can love another unconditionally, sacrificing for that person. But for that relationship to work, to be full of joy, the love has to go both ways. We'll discuss that later in more detail.

Healthy relationships, whether romantic or not, have this kind of self-giving love coming from both partners. This changes a relationship from a 50-50 arrangement to 100-100. Not 100-0, in which one person does all the work, but 100-100 where both partners give their all for the other.

You may have seen 50-50 relationships in action. "I'll do this for you, if you do that for me. I've done other things for you and you owe me." People like that are always keeping score. And usually the score is tilted in their favor. He may forget some of the great things she's done for him, but he places great importance on some trivial things that he's done.

"What do you mean, I don't do anything? I washed the dishes tonight, didn't I?"

"Well, you should. They're your dishes. You decided you wanted an ice cream sundae in the middle of the night."

"It was just because you didn't serve dessert with dinner."

"It was a rich meal anyway. I slaved over it. Not that you'd notice."

"Don't give me that. I work hard all day to put that food on the table."

"And I don't work hard?"

Both partners are convinced that they give 60 percent or more to this relationship, and they're not getting enough in return. But when they commit themselves to self-giving love, they aren't concerned about giving more than the other person because they're not keeping score. Their focus is on their commitment and what they can give. This frees them to appreciate what they're getting.

So that's the first thing to remember about healthy relationships. They are "best friendships," in which both partners communicate, trust, and honor each other, and are committed to a self-giving love with no requirement for payback.

CHAPTER THIRTEEN

Balance

ℰℐ

I MAGINE THIS. YOU WORK AS A BOAT-PERSON AT HARRY'S HONEYMOON Haven, a resort at one of the lakes near Niagara Falls. All sorts of couples come to the resort, which features an idyllic rowboat ride across the beautiful lake. It's your job to row the boat. The husband sits at one end, the wife at the other, and you're in the middle rowing. That's not the most romantic arrangement, but go with me on this—I'm making it up as I go along.

In your vast experience ferrying couples across the lake, you've had to deal with various issues of balance. Sometimes husbands are huge and wives are small, or vice versa. You compensate for this by moving slightly toward the lighter person, evening the load somewhat. There have been some challenges, but you've always been able to maintain balance on your boat.

Until you meet Big George Bumpus and his wife, Tiny.

You can sense there will be trouble. It's not that the weight differential is so great, but Big George has been drinking. His breath smells of whiskey and he keeps calling you "Ferdinand" for some odd reason, which apparently goes back to his bull-fighting days.

Big George staggers to your boat, flashing a wad of bills and insisting that you show him this lovely lake. You protest, but he's already in the boat, and you figure it would be more trouble to get him out. So you help Tiny into the small craft, position yourself on her side of the center, and row out toward the middle of the lake. So far, so good.

But then Big George starts to imagine things.

Mosquitoes the size of Brahma bulls, or something like that. In his unstable condition, he lurches to the side—and that does it. The boat capsizes. Only the life preserver and your own lifeguard training save Big George's life. Tiny swims safely to shore and is never seen again.

Relationships are like that. They find a certain equilibrium. We've all seen couples in which one partner seems stronger than the other. That's not necessarily bad.

Often one person will have a stronger personality; the other might be more submissive by nature. My friend Bill is like that. He is easy-going and soft-spoken, while his wife, Melanie, is a dynamo. She's vivacious and talented, full of ideas and energy. At first glance, you might think this relationship is seriously out of balance. How can he allow himself to be dominated like that? But as I've gotten to know Bill and Melanie, I've gained a great appreciation for the quality of their marriage. Bill doesn't say much, but when he speaks, Melanie pays attention. And he's comfortable with Melanie's exuberance. They complement each other. As long as both are giving love and nurturing the other, it's beautiful.

Even with disparate personalities, adjustments can be made to create a workable balance in a relationship—as we saw with the rowboat. But when one partner is out of balance personally, it threatens the balance of the relationship. That becomes an unhealthy situation—and dangerous. In the boat story, Big George had a problem. It wasn't Tiny's problem, except that she married him. It wasn't your problem, except that you were in the middle of a lake with him. His problem created a problem for the whole boat, just as one partner's personal problem creates a problem for the whole relationship. Healthy relationships are well-balanced, and the people within them are well-balanced.

Personal Balance

We are all collections of disparate elements. We are strong and weak. We are confident and insecure. We are extroverted and introverted.

I recently took one of those personality profile tests. That's where they ask you a bunch of questions, you tell them what you're like, and they turn around and tell you what you just told them. Brilliant!

I did like the fact that this particular test graded me on a scale. It didn't say, "You are a Feeler rather than a Thinker." It said, "You're about a 62 percent on the Feeler side of the Thinker-Feeler scale." That's an important difference because I am a thinker. I just tend to give my feelings priority—roughly 62 percent of the time.

As I said, each person is a combination of qualities. Personal balance comes from accepting *all* of who we are, the minority as well as the majority. I need to express my thinking side as well as my feeling side. It's a matter of wholeness. If I deny a part of who I am, I'm no longer whole.

Whole people keep work and play in proper perspective. They don't live for the weekend, but neither do they live at their jobs.

Whole people enjoy their family life, but they also have outside friends and they can be by themselves.

Whole people can set some ambitious goals for themselves, but they are aware of their own limitations. They push themselves at a reasonable rate.

Whole people give freely of themselves—their time, their concern, their resources—to others, but they also guard their own wholeness. They are aware when they're burning out. They can say no before they have no more to give.

Whole people can function independently of others, but they choose to make themselves somewhat dependent on those they love. They create an interdependence with others, on which good relationships are built.

Whole people are aware of their spirituality. They have a healthy relationship with God, but they also live out their faith in practical ways. They accept and enjoy the physicality of human life.

Whole people do not let addictions throw them out of balance. They avoid substance abuse because this would limit their capacities, making them less whole. They guard against other behavioral addictions, such as gambling or pornography, because these activities put artificial emphasis on one small aspect of a person and deny the rest.

Whole people can enjoy themselves in a variety of pleasurable pursuits, but they don't put undue importance on a momentary high. They look at the big picture of a satisfying lifestyle.

All of that may seem ideal to you. It may seem out of reach, unrealistic. But it's not. There are many well-balanced people around. I'm not talking about perfection; we all have our faults. But many people find an individual equilibrium and live in healthy ways. Others are moving toward that equilibrium.

Balance of Aspects

Relationships have various aspects: mental, spiritual, physical, social, personal. Relationships get out of balance when they focus on one of those aspects and ignore the others.

This happens most commonly with the physical aspect of a relationship. Our society prizes physical attraction; that's where most of our bonding starts. But how many couples have based their whole relationship on "you look great and you're good in bed"? They wake up one day and realize that they don't really *know* each other at all. Their personalities conflict, they don't think the same way, and they embarrass each other in public. It's out of balance.

Some might emphasize the social aspect of their relationship. They complement each other in public. People comment that they belong together, they're a great team. But get them alone and they can't stand each other. Or perhaps they have major spiritual or intellectual differences.

This is one thing I tell couples who are still dating. If you jump into physical involvement with each other, you are building an unbalanced relationship. You can't possibly know each other that intimately on a mental or spiritual level, but here you are zooming ahead with the physical. Slow down and grow together in all areas as you head toward a committed love. Keep things in balance.

There will always be those who are naturally more intellectual or more spiritually astute or more socially active. But in the best relationships, couples seek to strengthen the areas where they're naturally weak. They work at knowing each other in those other uncharted territories.

Balance Between Partners

Katie fell in love with Bob in college. He was witty and bright, and they thought alike on many things. They could talk together for hours. She felt she understood him better than others did, and she found his ideas stimulating.

After they dated for a while, Bob told Katie about a medical problem that sometimes affected his behavior. He was on medication, but she needed to understand his plight and allow for it. Now she understood him even better. Eventually they moved in together.

But Bob began to be quite demanding. He had a hard time finding and keeping a job. She encouraged him, typed resumes, scoured the want ads, and sent him out the door. When he did land a job, he would get bored with it in a few months.

In their relationship, whenever Bob did something wrong, he blamed it on his medical problem. Whenever he wanted something from her, he appealed to her sense of pity.

Through all of this, Katie felt unappreciated. Nobody was taking care of her. She realized that the relationship was out of balance. It was all about Bob and his problem. She was just there to help him cope. Feeling overwhelmed by him and his needs, she asked him to move out, though they would continue to date.

As a painter, she had an opportunity to show some paintings at a gallery in a distant city. She traveled there for the opening, a major event in her life and career. To her dismay, Bob didn't call to wish her luck before she left. When he did call, four days after she returned, he talked about what he had been doing. Nothing about her trip. That was the end of that relationship. She broke up with him shortly afterward, and he couldn't understand why.

Katie was more than willing to give Bob the care and support he needed. But she needed something in return. The relationship was dangerously out of balance, and that was throwing her out of balance personally. She was wise to get out of it.

A healthy relationship is not about him, it's not about her—it's about *them*. Partners recognize certain times when one may need to support the other, but there's a healthy give and take, and the balance is restored soon afterward. In public, they talk about each other, and they use the words "us" and "we" a lot. (Out-of-balance relationships usually have one partner saying "me" a lot and the other saying "him" or "her.")

It may be that one partner has a better job, is more outgoing, or is a natural leader. And the other partner may naturally move into a support role. If both are satisfied with that arrangement, there's nothing wrong with it. But for good balance to be maintained, they still need to think of themselves as a team fulfilling different roles on the team—not as "her supporting him" or vice versa.

Earlier I talked about keeping score. There are different ways of doing this. When couples are in trouble, they start to play a zero-sum game. That is, if I get ahead, you must be behind. What's good for me is bad for you. You might see that as a kind of "balance," but it's not good.

For the past several years, the Chicago Bulls have dominated pro basketball. Their two finest players are Michael Jordan and Scottie Pippen, both perennial all-stars. These guys regularly score twenty or thirty points a game, but one night Jordan leads the scoring, and the next night Pippen has the hit hand. It would be absurd for them to compete against each other, except maybe in fun. They're on the same team! What's good for Jordan is good for Pippen, and they know it. That's why you see Jordan driving to the basket, drawing the defenders, and dishing off to Pippen for an easy slam.

Healthy relationships are like that. Both partners know they're on the same team. They work to support and encourage and inspire each other.

There's no zero-sum game there. Good relationships, even among competitive people, have that aspect of encouragement, challenge, and inspiration. When one wins, both win. That's the kind of balance a healthy relationship requires.

Chapter Fourteen

Boundaries

❧

"MY BOYFRIEND USED TO SLAP ME AROUND. WAS I SUPPOSED TO LOVE him unconditionally, in spite of that physical abuse?"

The woman was responding to a talk given at a Fresh Start seminar for separated and divorced people. My colleague Tom Jones had just spoken about unconditional love, which "looks for nothing in return, but gives, gives, gives."

Tom does a great job with that subject, but he often gets a heated response.

"I did give, give, give," one man complained, "and I got nothing in return. Now I'm a mess."

"I let my husband use me for years," a woman added, "and then he ran off with someone else."

"That unconditional love stuff sounds good," one person piped up, "but it just doesn't fly." The others nodded agreement.

Tom urged them to return for my talk later in the day on the subject of boundaries. Soon after that, we switched the order of the talks. People need to understand boundaries before they can practice unconditional love.

Unconditional love is a personal ideal. As an individual, you need to offer love with no selfish strings attached.

Otherwise, it's not love, just manipulation or bargaining.

Loving friends is easy because you know you'll get something back. But treating people with love when they're acting unlovable. . . well, that's a trick. They may sneer at you or spit on you or slap you around. To show love in those circumstances is a supreme challenge, though it *can* be done.

In a relationship, new rules enter the picture. Suddenly I must be concerned not only with you and me, but with us. I may live my life in a self-giving, undemanding, sacrificial way. I may give my coat to the panhandler on the corner and my last dollar to the Salvation Army. But for a relationship to work, the love has to flow *both* ways. For the good of "us," I must require you to show love to me as well. That takes boundaries.

Poet Robert Frost was onto something profound in his poem "Mending Wall," in which he wrote, "Good fences make good neighbors." We tend to think that everything in a relationship should be free and open. No secrets, no closed doors, no boundaries. We don't like walls—but they are necessary for good relationships. Good fences make good partners.

I had a landlady who held a grudge against the guy next door because she had been mowing one strip of grass that belonged to that neighbor for ten years and never got a thank-you. My landlady was a gem. She would bring me food and pick up my mail when I was out of town. She was a giving person, but she was nasty toward the neighbor. All over one strip of grass.

"Maybe he thinks it belongs to you," I suggested once, and the thought stunned my landlady for a moment. Then she shook her head—no, no, that couldn't be.

They could have used a fence, a boundary. Then they would have known what was required and what was extra. They would have known the rules.

Any relationship between a man and a woman is a trinity—he, she, and it. It's a three-legged stool. In order to have an "it" (the relationship), you need both a "he" and a "she." If they lose themselves, if they don't know who they are, if the relationship becomes exclusively about one partner or the other—the stool collapses. All three are necessary. How can you ensure that all three will be strong? You need to protect your own self, empower your partner, and define the relationship.

Protecting Your Self

Picture this. A person walks inside on a hot day, gets a pitcher of water out of the refrigerator, and pours it—all over the kitchen table. Without a glass to hold the water, it's pretty useless—it's all over the place. The water needs boundaries. That's just the way liquid is.

So it is with a person. Some people "pour themselves out" for their partners. They lose all sense of who they are. Their whole identity is wrapped up in the other person. They have no boundaries. Sad to say, those people are like the water dripping onto the kitchen floor. Without those personal boundaries, they can't do much good—even for the people they're pouring themselves out for.

Bonnie was like that. You remember her story: going as a missionary to France, only to be used by her husband, then used by another man, and another. She gave up her personal boundaries. With low self-esteem to begin with, she kept trying to find her worth in these men. She served them. She made herself of use to them (and then complained that they "used" her).

There are many people like this, so devoted to their partners that they ditch their moral convictions, give up their rights, sever their friendships, quit their jobs, change their religion, and more. They give up everything that makes them uniquely "them" in order to merge more closely with their partners.

How do you know if you are lacking "personal boundaries"? Symptoms may include the following:

- Being unable to keep secrets
- Talking at an intimate level on the first date

- Falling in love at first sight
- Falling in love with anyone who shows interest
- Thinking about someone all the time
- Violating your personal sexual standards
- Accepting food, gifts, or touching that you don't want
- Feeling that your opinion doesn't matter
- Running yourself ragged for someone else's sake (especially when they aren't lifting a finger)
- Letting others make decisions for you
- Letting others tell you how you feel
- Letting a partner decide who your friends will be
- Losing control so someone will take care of you
- Putting up with sexual or physical abuse
- Feeling obligated to do things for people you hardly know
- Finding it hard to say no, even when you know you should

It's not selfish to draw the line. You have to say, "Wait a second! This is who I am. I have certain rules, certain convictions, certain friends, certain requirements. I'll meet you halfway. I'll even go more than halfway, but you need to honor me for who I am."

We've seen this self-awareness in the cases of Sally and Laurie. They were able to grab the reins of their own identity and to determine that they were worth more than they thought. They didn't need to sink themselves into addictive relationships. They could be worthy people as individuals.

We sometimes talk about people being "users." They want other people to serve them, to make their lives easier. Often people with low self-esteem (and no personal boundaries) become "usees." And guess what? Usees attract users.

Karen told me, "I am a magnet for bad men." That's truer than she knows. As long as she operates without boundaries, seeking to serve every man she meets in any way she can, she'll scare away the good men and attract the bad. It's a sad fact.

If people who are being used in relationships were to stand up and declare their personal boundaries, it often would put an end to those relationships. The users would not respect those new boundaries. They'd be off looking for someone else to use. That might be hard for the usee to take, but it's probably the best thing.

When I talk about boundaries, however, I'm not talking about rigid definitions. It's not "That's the way I am and I'm not going to change; take it or leave it, baby." Obviously, healthy relationships have some give and take. Your partner will affect you deeply, and you will affect your partner. To extend the liquid analogy, you might want to think of your "container" as a plastic bag full of water. It adapts to outside pressure, but it still contains and defines the liquid inside.

Empowering Your Partner

In the language of addiction and codependency, we often speak of enablers. These are the people—often a spouse or significant other—who help an addicted person to manage his or her addiction. Sounds great, doesn't it? It's not. The enabler actually helps the addict stay addicted.

When Sally's kids called in sick for her, they were enabling. Sure, they were just trying to help. Mom needed to keep her job. But they were making it possible, at least for a while, for Sally to maintain her addictions and still lead a rather normal life. And that kept Sally from seeking the help she needed—until it was almost too late.

Enablers make up for the effects of an addict's addiction. Enablers make excuses for the addict. Enablers are always forgiving, always trusting. They are often drawn into the addiction themselves.

What if you're not dealing with an alcohol or drug problem? Can enabling still occur? In a way, yes. If your relationship is out of balance, if you would describe it as addictive, if you are being used by a user, you may be enabling your partner to treat you in unsatisfactory ways.

One client of mine regularly waited a half-hour, an hour, or more for her partner to show up for a date. Every time she forgave him and agreed to go out with him again, she was enabling him to continue his inconsiderate tardiness.

But shouldn't you forgive? Yes, you should, but you should also hold your partner accountable for his or her behavior. Remember that three-legged stool. You can forgive everything between "he" and "she" but the offending partner needs to know that the misdeed has harmed "it"—the relationship. The rules have been broken. The relationship will not survive long if that behavior continues, even if you offer personal forgiveness for any pain you sustained.

As I see it, the alternative to enabling is *empowering*. Instead of enabling your partner to continue in bad ways, you seek to empower your partner to conquer those bad ways. That empowering happens not through excuses but encounters, not through forgive and forget, but forgive and remind (of the rules of the relationship).

This is a dangerous concept because you can only take it so far. You will not "save" your partner. If the relationship becomes all about teaching your partner how to treat you right, you're losing balance. The point is that by playing hardball with an errant partner, you may challenge him or her to change. Or you may not.

Empowering means saying to your partner, "You are worth more than this. You are capable of better behavior." If your partner is caught up in some self-destructive addiction, you want to help that person recognize his or her value, and you want not to destroy but restore. But relationships can be self-destructive as well, for both partners. If there is physical or mental abuse, the abuser is also abusing his own soul. Empowering is not saving, but issuing a challenge rooted in the value of that person.

Defining the Relationship

Somewhere along the line, you need to decide what kind of a relationship you're going to have. This simple piece of advice may seem obvious, but many couples trip over it. I know guys who got married, expecting their wives to do the housewife routine, only to find that their wives were planning careers of their own. A guy like that wants to bring home the bacon and be sure his wife cooks it. He doesn't expect a life full of microwave dinners.

They need to talk about who they are, what they want, what they need from each other. They need to define their relationship.

I talked with Rob about some of the frustrations in his dating life. "I was dating this one woman—she was great—though it was still very casual between us," he said. "She had this bad habit of canceling out on dates at the last minute. I'd find a message on the answering machine saying she couldn't make it and she'd call later to explain. Well, she wouldn't call. So a week or two later I'd call her again and she'd be all nice and everything, and we'd go out a few times. And then she'd cancel again.

"We went through that whole cycle twice. Then one night I went to pick her up for a date and she wasn't there.

"I was knocking at her door, with fifty-dollar tickets in my pocket, and she wasn't there. That's when I decided I'd had enough. She was gorgeous, but I guess she knew it. I just couldn't let her treat me like that."

By going through the cycle twice, Rob and this woman were "defining their relationship" like this: She can cancel out at the last minute and that's okay because Rob will forgive her and ask her out again. Those aren't good terms for a relationship. By refusing to call her now, Rob is protesting those terms. If she wants to go out with him, she'll have to follow through on her commitments.

David, from our original circle, told me how he was stringing along a young woman he was dating. She was crazy about him, and he was so-so about her. Then one day she erupted into a

"You don't bring me flowers" speech. She was feeling unloved and unappreciated. She was trying to redefine the relationship: "I regularly show you how much I care for you, David, and you don't show me anything in return. That has to change."

It changed for a while, but David realized that he did not want to have that kind of relationship with this woman. Ultimately, he broke up with her. That caused her some pain, but it was far better than being strung along in an undefined, ill-defined relationship. She forced his hand, defined her terms, and eventually freed herself from a potentially addictive relationship.

How do you do this? How can you define a relationship you're in?

1. Decide what you need from the relationship and what you're willing to give. I don't want to make it sound too much like corporate negotiations, but you need to be prepared.

2. Talk with your partner. Start by asking what he or she wants from you in this relationship. Your partner may not know. Or there may be things under the surface that are not mentioned outright.

3. Discuss with your partner what you need. See if you have any unreasonable requests (or if your partner does).

4. If necessary, draw up an agreed set of "rules" for the relationship. If your relationship is already in pretty good shape, the communication of the first three steps may be enough. But if things have to change, agree together on the terms of your relationship. Bringing flowers. Being on time. Not canceling dates at the last minute. Doing some things that you want to do. Going out with your friends sometimes.

Or there may be more serious issues. Stop hitting me. Stop doing drugs. Cool it on the sexual relationship. Don't belittle me in public.

5. Be ready to leave if the rules are not followed. Decide in advance: One strike? Two strikes? Three? How important are those rules to you? Are you willing to live by these relationship boundaries?

6. Be aware that the relationship may not survive.

This is not just playing games. If you hold to certain boundaries, your partner may leave you, as David left the woman who wanted more from him. You may find that someone you want doesn't want you badly enough to play by your rules, as Rob discovered. That may be painful for the moment, but it's the best thing for you.

It's also possible that your partner will respond positively. You might restore your relationship on healthy, equitable terms. And that, of course, would be good, too.

⅏

SO what does a healthy relationship look like when it has good boundaries? Both partners are aware of what they need from the other, as well as what they need to give. They communicate freely when they are especially needy or feel used.

As best friends, they are willing to give 60, 90, or even 100 percent, but they also know that the relationship needs to be in balance. Each partner learns to lean on the other and to be leaned on.

The "good fences" are there, but you'd hardly know it. There is no nitpicking, just a fair distribution of effort and love.

CHAPTER FIFTEEN

Case Study: Christine

༆

CHRISTINE WAS ALWAYS A GOOD GIRL. "QUIET AND GOOD," SHE SAYS, looking back on her childhood. Christine was an only child, but didn't get the attention that usually goes with that status. Her father worked hard to care for her mother, who was frequently ill, and to pay the medical bills. Christine stayed in the background, quiet and good, wanting to be of help, but not sure what to do. She overheard an aunt say that Christine's birth may have intensified her mother's illness.

Her mother died when she was twelve.

By then, her father didn't know how to deal with her. He continued to work hard and paid little attention to Christine.

Marriage and Afterward

Christine married a man very much like her father. Oh, at the time she thought he was gloriously different, but soon she fell into the same routine. He was a workaholic, she says, and she stayed home, quiet and good, eager to please, craving his attention. They were married twelve years, and he never knew where anything was in the kitchen. That was her domain.

Then he had an affair and left her. The man she had served for a dozen years, and dated six years before that, was gone.

Two years later, she found a new man. This man was different, she thought. He was needy. He had been divorced only two weeks—his wife had just up and left—and he had a twelve-year-old daughter. Christine could identify with this girl who had just lost her mother. "I wanted to take care of her," she says simply. And the girl's father, John, needed caring, too.

Christine slid into her old role, giving and forgiving, quiet and good. John was frequently late for dates—anywhere from a half-hour to four hours late—and he wouldn't call. Christine was irked, but she put up with it. "He always had excuses. He said he didn't have a watch, so I bought him one. He wouldn't wear it. And he'd still be late."

Like her father and like her husband, John was unavailable. He worked nights and weekends. Even when he was physically present, he wasn't emotionally with her. Christine was frustrated by this, but this was all she had ever known. She was fighting the same old fight, struggling to win attention from a father figure.

John was restless. He said he wanted to date others. "Fine," said Christine. But he didn't. They dated for four years and then got engaged. John was still restless.

"I'm not ready to get married again," he would say. Not ready? After four years? But he was right. He hooked up with Christine so soon after his divorce that there were still too many personal issues unresolved. Life was so easy with Christine serving him hand and foot—but was that what he really wanted?

Finally John broke the engagement. He began dating someone else, whom he eventually married.

Trying Again

A year later, Christine fell in love again. "He walked through my front door and my heart fell to the floor," she says. She had never believed in "love at first sight," but this was it.

New man, same story. "He was much like my ex-husband: emotionally unavailable. I have never seen anyone stay in depression for that long." They dated for two years and broke up.

"In every relationship I have," she says, "I seem to go after someone who won't give me the attention I want. They're all unavailable in some way. I keep thinking it's me, that I have a problem, but I'm realizing that they just don't have it in them. That's the kind of man I choose."

Experts have suggested that when people look for mates, they often look for people like their parents—and try to change them. The childhood battles are fought all over again. This is true in Christine's case and in many others' lives. The "unavailable man syndrome" is common. Our society has groomed a generation of men who don't know how to give of themselves. Women like Christine get frustrated by this, but they give in to it. Their only strategy for success is to be "quiet and good" and servile and forgiving. They lose all personal boundaries and allow themselves to be taken for granted.

Seeking an Answer

After this last two-year relationship, Christine went to see a female colleague of mine. Her presenting problem was actually a food addiction. In the wake of this latest romantic failure, she was eating to numb her feelings. The counselor was able to confront the relationship addiction that was eating at her.

They began to talk about the kind of man Christine was attracted to. She has a natural attraction to good-looking men, but there was something else, too. She gravitates toward men who are emotionally unavailable. "If I'm immediately attracted to someone," she says, "I know there must be something terribly wrong with him." It's as if she longs for that challenge.

With her counselor's help, Christine has tried to change her ways. "I'm still probably going to have the tendencies," she says. "I'm still probably going to be attracted to the wrong people. But

I'm learning not to judge a man for a potential relationship merely on the basis of whether I'm attracted to him. If I think he's a nice person and has a few marbles right in his head, I'll try to get to know him better."

As she does get to know a man, Christine has learned to focus on how he acts—not on how he looks or what he says. "Look at his life," she tells herself. "How does he conduct himself?" She can sniff out a workaholic at ten paces. And she's learning to sense when a man is in denial about underlying problems. (That was the problem with John, who probably hadn't dealt with the deep-felt issues of his divorce. He was comfortable with Christine, but needed to do some difficult soul-searching before he could move on with a new relationship.)

Christine also has learned to establish good patterns at the beginning of a relationship. Shortly after she began counseling, she met a man who seemed interesting. She wasn't physically attracted to him, but he was intelligent and kind. Under her new rules, she decided to try to get to know him better.

She expressed interest, and they went out a few times. She was very careful not to be too servile, as was her habit. "I gave nothing," she says, almost proudly. "If anything, I was too demanding." But she drew some affirmation from the fact that he enjoyed her company. He liked Christine for who she was, not for the things she could do for him.

He was honest about the fact that he was dating someone else as well. That was fine. Christine was determined to go slowly with this relationship. Ironically, the other woman gave him an ultimatum—all or nothing—and he decided to stop dating Christine.

There was none of the deep pain of previous breakups. Christine had kept this relationship under control. She had successfully played by her new rules.

A few weeks later, the guy called back. "Maybe I made a mistake. I really miss you. Maybe we could go out again." What would the old Christine have said—the one with no boundaries? "Sure! Whatever! I'm here for you!"

But now Christine was friendly but firm: "When you make up your mind, call me."

Christine also learned to consult her friends and her counselor for advice about new relationships. She has a close friend whose dating life has paralleled her own. She now seeks this friend's opinion. It also helped to be accountable to her counselor. This kept her from "love at first sight" attractions. Those things are great for the movies, but in real life they're fraught with difficulties.

As with so many relationship addictions, in Christine's case it comes down to self-image issues. Her troubles have stemmed from a fuzzy sense of who she is. If she's not gaining attention from a man, what good is she? She is learning that she has tremendous value all by herself. After a lot of work in counseling, she now says, "I think I deserve the best. I'm not going to settle."

A Breakthrough

Christine made a breakthrough when she restored her relationship with her father. They had seen each other on rare occasions, but Christine's counselor urged her to see her father again and try to resolve those issues of paternal love and attention-seeking.

They had lunch together, and Christine poured out her soul. It was awkward—a man who had never been good at expressing his feelings, and a woman for whom he was still somehow responsible. Christine told of her failed relationships and the pain of each one. She was trying to be nice about it, but she could not be the "quiet and good" child any longer.

"One of the problems is," she stammered, "I think it comes down to . . . you never said you loved me."

Her father squirmed in his seat. "Of course I did," he shrugged. "I mean, I do." At the time, Christine wasn't sure how much to trust that grudging confession. But as they got up to leave,

Christine's father moved over to her awkwardly and embraced her. "I really do love you," he said.

There was great healing in that moment. Christine has continued to meet with her father for lunch. And she continues to meet with her counselor. She is putting her life back together—on her terms.

Evaluation

Once again, we see a childhood drama played out into adulthood. Christine's distant relationship with her father clearly affected her relations with men. She engaged in a form of self-sabotage by subconsciously seeking out men who were like her father. This type of man held an attraction for her, a challenge. And of course there are many men like that out there, willing to be served, but unavailable emotionally.

The food addiction is an interesting sidelight.

Christine describes it as a "numbing" thing. Her sensations of emotional pain over the constant rejection of the men she wants are overcome by the pleasant sensations of taste. There may be some self-sabotage there, too.

The outlook for Christine is good. She has been "finding herself," establishing a solid self-image. She has been disciplining herself with food and with men, regaining control of her desires. She has re-examined her priorities, re-evaluating what she really wants in a man. And the renewed contact with her father is tremendously healing. It will not make all the childhood pain disappear, but it will salve those wounds. Over time, this paternal relationship can help renew and restore Christine's sense of self.

One final note on these case studies: I have presented people in various situations. Some are in the middle of their struggles. They may have taken some steps toward recovery, but there's a long road ahead. Others, you might say, are healed. Their lives are back together. They seem healthy and happy.

Yet even these "healthy people" know they could easily slip

back to their addictive ways. They're like the recovering drug or alcohol abusers who continue to describe themselves as "recovering" years later. Their attitude is: "I'm back on track now, but I know what I need to guard against. I will continue to be careful."

Such caution is best for all of us, but it's especially important for those who are prone to unbalanced relationships. With caution, they can recover, and they can develop healthy new relationships.

CHAPTER SIXTEEN

Addiction Within a Marriage

𝔭𝔞

PEOPLE IN ADDICTIVE RELATIONSHIPS OFTEN GET MARRIED. NATURALLY, they carry into the marriage all the controlling, jealousy, manipulation, obsession, abuse, and low self-esteem they had before the marriage. Often they think marriage will solve these problems. It doesn't. It creates new problems and limits their options — specifically the option to walk away from the relationship.

Another psychologist told me of a couple she had been counseling, a classic case of addictions run wild. Both had serious self-esteem issues in their backgrounds. Both had serious needs. Both had been through failed marriages and maintained custody of their children.

Their romance was quickly intimate. It was their children who first recognized the danger. Both partners were losing themselves in this new relationship — it was not healthy. Still, they were headed toward marriage. They consulted my colleague for premarital counseling.

One more thing: Both partners had tempers. It didn't take much to set them off. Their counselor found it hard to keep up. In one session they'd be cooing over each other, and in the next they'd curse and spit. These weren't just lovers' spats, either; these were out-and-out, I-never-want-to-see-you-again, I-despise-the-ground-you-walk-on brawls. But after a few weeks apart, they had to see each other, and they'd be back at it.

This love-hate cycle is a hallmark of addictive relationships. Driven by a compulsion to be with each other, they bring out the worst in each other and antagonize each other. Neither one is growing or helping the other grow. They seek relief for their deep emotional needs, but instead they reopen old wounds. It's "I'm nobody if you don't love me" but "you only love me for about a day or so before finding something terribly wrong with me."

Finally, in private sessions, both admitted it was an unhealthy addictive relationship, and they should cool it while they worked on their own emotional needs. Good plan—except that within a month they were engaged to be married. "We just couldn't stand to be apart," they said.

Did the marriage change anything? What do you think? The last time I spoke with their counselor, she said they'd been fighting frequently. And in their first year of marriage, one or the other had moved out three different times.

The addictive dating relationship had become an addictive marriage. Marrying each other served only to close the back door. It added new ropes to tie them together. It made it much more difficult for them to find the individual healing each of them needed.

The Exception

Every rule has its exceptions. I've been telling you that "cold turkey" is the way to go: If you are in an addictive relationship, get out. But here's the one exception, and it's a huge one. If you are married, try as hard as you can to keep the marriage together.

You see, though I believe that relationship addicts need to stay away from the objects of their addiction, I believe even more in the sanctity of marriage. I take those vows seriously. In the wedding ceremony, we promise to be loyal "till death do us part" (or whatever they're saying nowadays). That's an oath to God and to each other. It's not "till I no longer feel fulfilled in this relationship" or "until my partner does something really bad."

I understand that we're not talking about casual divorce: "Oh, I'm bored with this one; let me try a new spouse." I understand that we're talking about emotional health, and that's serious. This is a very tough call, but I don't know how I can say anything other than this: If you're married, you've made a commitment to stay with that marriage.

I know many people who are enduring difficult marriages. Personalities aren't clicking anymore. Arguments abound. Each day is a struggle. I admire their tenacity, their desire to stay together even when it doesn't seem worth it. If that's your situation—trapped in an unhealthy, addictive marriage—this chapter is a challenge. You have the unenviable task of climbing back up that slope, trying to regain your balance and your boundaries, and restoring the health of your relationship. Of course, many of the principles you've already read in this book will apply to your situation, but this chapter should offer some extra insight.

Detachment

Earlier I mentioned addiction as a matter of attaching. We attach our own significance, identity, or pleasure to someone or something. Gerald May points out that our word *attach* comes from a French word meaning "nailed to." He comments, "Attachment 'nails' our desire to specific objects and creates addiction."[1] If you are addicted to a specific person, think of yourself as "nailed" to him or her. That person can't do a thing without you caring or worrying or responding or wondering what he or she thinks about you. Everything you do is somehow nailed to that person as well. Will your partner approve? Will your partner notice? How does it compare to what your partner does? Will it make your partner happy?

You can see that in the case of the fighting couple I just described. Even when they couldn't stand each other, they were obsessed with each other. Every action that one of them did was viewed as a statement to the other. In that context, a raised eyebrow, a yawn, or a certain tone of voice ("What did you mean by that?") can spark an argument.

They were clearly attached to each other, nailed tight, and the marriage just pounded in a few more nails.

Attachment is common among codependents (which is why the literature of Al-Anon and similar groups refers to it frequently). A codependent attaches his or her own sense of significance to the welfare of the addicted partner. Every rise and fall in the addict's recovery deeply affects the codependent partner. The codependent's well-being is nailed to that of the addict. This creates caretaking situations in which the codependent makes decisions for the addict and thus limits the addict's responsibility. It also leads to enabling behavior in which the codependent helps the addict manage the addiction and still lead a nearly normal life. The codependent may think he or she is just serving the best interests of the addicted partner, but at that level of attachment there is no distinction. Their interests are nailed together.

If you find yourself in an addictive marriage, you need to begin a process of *detachment*. In severe cases, this might mean an actual separation, but that's not what I have in mind. (In cases of physical abuse, I do recommend immediate separation. Abuse cannot be tolerated.) I'm talking about an emotional detachment, a process of finding yourself and releasing your partner.

Ideally, this will free you both for personal growth so you can come together later on healthier terms. At the least, it will help you in your personal growth and keep you from going down the tubes of a bad relationship.

Detachment is based on the belief that each person is responsible for him or herself. We can't solve problems that aren't ours to solve, and we can't make someone else change. We adopt a policy of keeping our hands off other people's responsibilities and tending to our own areas of weakness.

When people create problems for themselves, we need to allow them to face the consequences of their actions. We allow people to be who they are. It's their responsibility to grow, mature, and develop. We in turn accept our own responsibility for personal growth.

If we can't solve a problem and we've done all we could, we learn to live with, or in spite of, that problem. Then we try to live happily, focusing heroically on what is good in our lives today and feeling grateful for that. We learn the important lesson that making the most of what we have multiplies our blessings.

Darla

Let me tell you about one of those "heroes," my friend Darla. She'd probably say she hasn't done anything especially courageous, but I think she has. Darla is in the process of detaching from her husband, for her own growth and sanity, but she isn't divorcing him. She has weathered some hard times and still has a bad marriage, but there's now a glimmer of hope.

Darla met Stan at church about six years ago.

Both were in their thirties, divorced, and emotionally needy. Nothing was working out for Stan. He couldn't keep a job, and he had various business schemes that always seemed to fail. Darla loved his vulnerability. He was open and honest with her then. She, a caretaker by nature, had found someone to take care of.

They were great friends then. Only after friends suggested they'd make a great couple did they begin to consider a romance. After a lengthy friendship, they had a fairly short courtship. They already knew each other pretty well—or so they thought.

Both suffered from low self-esteem. He was rather bright, in a street-smart way, but a learning disability had kept him from going to college. Each new business disappointment rankled him and stabbed at his pride. He bragged that he had learned far more in life than most people learn in college. He complained that the world was prejudiced against those without formal education. But his words masked a deep insecurity. Darla tended to agree with him, though she was college-educated and had credits toward an MBA. She saw his brilliance in a way few others did. She could be his savior.

As you can see, there were some elements of an addictive relationship from the start. It was already a bit out of balance. The relationship was largely about him—helping him get on his feet economically, helping him unlock his potential. And Darla was more than happy to function this way.

Stan and Darla married and had children. She helped him start a business, and it prospered. They were able to buy a nice house in a nice community, and he began to hobnob with the business leaders of the community. Then there were other businesses he started, with some successes and some failures. Still, each failure stabbed at Stan; he had a lot to prove.

Darla noticed that Stan spent more and more time at his job. He was obsessed with his work. At home, he was too tired to do much of anything. He took up golf and became obsessed with that, spending most of his weekends improving his game.

He was suddenly distant. They never talked as they used to. He didn't go out with Darla, nor did he help with the kids or the house. When Darla complained, he became extremely defensive. He claimed he was still more communicative, more emotional, more vulnerable than most men, but then he'd pack up his things for a trip to some faraway golf haven. He worked hard, very hard, for Darla and the kids, he argued. He needed golf to unwind after a hard week of work.

It was as if he were protecting some precious treasure within, and Darla couldn't be trusted with it.

At first, Darla denied the problem. Surely Stan was just going through a rough time, right? The crisis would blow over, right?

No. The problem continued and Darla had to handle it. She worked closely with Stan in one of his business ventures in an effort to enter his world. Maybe he would open up to her in that venue. It didn't happen. The tension carried over to the work-place, so Darla quit. Soon afterward she earned her MBA and got a low-level business job in the city.

Then she got angry. The more she thought about it, the angrier she got. How dare he treat her like that! How dare he put his job—and golf, for goodness, sake!—ahead of his family. He was a tightwad with the family, always claiming that money was tight, but then he'd fly off on expensive weekend trips. She could never figure that out—and it made her mad. Yet whenever her anger erupted, he just closed up more and became more defensive. He nearly left her at this point. Her anger was not saving this marriage.

So then depression hit her, physically as well as emotionally. She lost a lot of weight and couldn't sleep. "The whole thing is something like learning to live with cancer," she says, tracing the pattern of denial, bargaining, anger, and depression. "Eventually you have to accept that this is the situation and I need to respond to it in a healthy way."

Darla came out of her depression, although her anger still simmers from time to time. But she's done a good job of redeeming a bad situation. She works hard and tries to be a good mother and wife. She keeps the lines of communication open with her husband but doesn't pressure him. She is, in many respects, an independent woman. She has learned to fend for herself, to live her own life. She even entertains friends at home—he's invited to join them, but often he begs off.

There's a glimmer of hope in the counseling they're both receiving. At least he has agreed to that. And there are faint signs that he is opening up. Darla has learned not to expect a lot. She knows there's a long, hard road ahead, but maybe things will change someday.

Surviving

If you find yourself being drawn into a downward spiral, it's essential that you detach yourself from it. Break free. Let me repeat that I'm not talking about divorce, though detachment may create distance. You are creating boundaries, walls that will protect your own existence. You are moving to higher ground and challenging your partner to join you there.

It's not easy. Your partner probably won't like it. Your spouse may divorce you. But you must maintain a vision of wholeness—for yourself and for your relationship—that will keep you going.

Everything must be done with love. As you begin to break free, you'll be tempted to hate, hurt, heckle, hound. But put all of that aside. Act in love. It's a sober, tough love that creates distance between husband and wife. It's a prayerful, vigilant love that seeks healing for the relationship on healthy terms. It's a difficult love, but it's strong love.

So how do you accomplish this? How can you "pull backward a bit" or "detach" from a bad situation? Besides the guidelines we've already mentioned throughout the book, here are some additional principles which may help you in your struggle.

1. Let go of your own self-destructive impulses. Each of us has certain buttons that, when pushed, launch us into an orbit of self-hate. It doesn't take our spouses long to find out where these are. We each have things we feel embarrassed or insecure about. Some of us have certain temptations we find hard to resist.

When someone says the wrong thing, we fight, sulk, feel guilty, lose our resolve, eat, smoke, tumble back into a bad relationship. We respond in different ways, but most of us are easily manipulated, especially by those closest to us.

You need to guard those buttons as carefully as if they launched nuclear warheads. Be ready with some self-talk to keep you out of orbit: "I will not feel guilty about that because I've been forgiven"; "I will not fight about this, it's not worth it"; "I am not responsible for this person's life."

Recognize your partner's statement (or action) for what it is, a conscious or subconscious attempt to manipulate you, to reel you in, to maintain the relationship at its old addictive level. Don't let it happen. You are beyond that now. You're on a mission. You can let go of all that personal baggage now because "winning" in this relationship isn't important anymore. You're moving on to a new game.

2. Let go of your expectations—but verbalize your needs. Darla told me of a time when she was taking night classes once a week. She left Stan home with the kids. You might think that when she got home the kids would already be put to bed and the place tidied up a bit. That's what she expected. But it never happened. The kids were clamoring, there were crumbs all over the couch, and Stan was sprawled out watching TV. She even dropped not-so-subtle hints about how she'd like Stan to put the kids to bed. Still, nothing happened.

Eventually, she had to let those expectations go. Stan would never do what she wanted in this matter; she had to accept that. In letting those expectations go, she released herself from the continual disappointment she had been feeling. She became angry and then depressed each time Stan failed her. She didn't need those feelings.

But she continued to verbalize her wishes and needs. She did not shut him out entirely. If he wanted to run this marriage on reasonable terms, she was always ready to let him know what she desired. She would try not to nag him, but she would still communicate.

Holding it inside and pretending it didn't bother her also would be wrong. She needed to learn the balance of letting go of her expectations, while verbalizing her needs. As she said, "Stuffing it only made me more angry and depressed."

At a church retreat for couples, spouses were asked to present each other with a "wish," something they'd like their partner to do for them. Darla wished to be taken out for dinner—even to McDonald's—or for an evening walk around the city—just the two of them. Stan agreed to do this sometime. She's still waiting. She brought it up a few weeks later. He grumbled something about not being able to afford a babysitter, and then he went out to buy some new golf clubs.

Darla has learned to accept this. She continues to present her wishes from time to time but refuses to get bent out of shape when they don't come true. (Perhaps you can see why I consider her attitude to be heroic.)

3. Let go of your control of your partner. This is crucial, especially if you're a caretaker by nature. In that case, a substantial part of your own identity is wrapped up in your partner's need for you. You regularly try to control, change, improve, or affect your mate's behavior. Your relationship may be largely based on that activity. And that's part of the problem.

Even if you're sure you are changing your mate for the better, you need to let go. Even if you fear your partner will fall apart without your control, you need to give up that control. You are not responsible for your mate. And as long as you control his or her behavior, your partner doesn't have to take responsibility for his or her own life. It is best for both of you if you stop controlling.

M. Scott Peck, author of the book *The Road Less Traveled*, echoed these thoughts when he reflected on much of the marriage counseling he has done over the years. "The problem with many couples is not too much separateness, but rather too much togetherness," he said in a lecture, going on to explain that a healthy relationship for those who are out of balance is many times a matter of "backing away from each other." He shared with the crowd that about five years into his own marriage, he and his wife "hit bottom." He got angry with his wife, began to withdraw from her, and finally started to not care about her so much. She reciprocated by not caring about him.

As Dr. Peck put it, "You know what I mean when I say we stopped caring about each other? I mean that I gave up trying to change and control her life, and she gave up trying to change or control me; and our marriage has been steadily improving ever since!"[2]

This concept reminds me of a children's toy I ran across years ago. It's a cylinder made from flexible interwoven strips called

Chinese handcuffs. If you put your fingers in on both sides and pull as hard as you can, it tightens and you can't get out. Only when you push in does it relax its grip. There are many relationships in which people are trapped because they're pulling so hard in one direction. "If only you become what I want you to be, we can have a great relationship." Even though they mean well, their desperate attempts to control the other person are trapping them in a bad situation. But when they relax, allowing the other person to make his or her own choices, they can escape from the grip of that relationship addiction.

It sounds easy, but of course it's very hard when you're in the middle of it. It would be one thing to walk away from the relationship, but to stay in the marriage and renounce your control—that's a challenge. You need to keep a check on your attitudes.

- "I will care about my spouse but I will not be a caretaker."
- "I will inspire but I will not enable."
- "I will communicate without nagging."
- "I will be humble but not self-destructive."
- "I will have a servant's heart but I will observe certain healthy boundaries."
- "I will allow my mate to disagree with me if he or she chooses; I will not give in just to keep the peace."

Darla found that her efforts to improve her relationship with Stan were met with more defensiveness. She was there with her college education (and a minor in psychology) trying to define the relationship on her terms. He resented her attempts to control things. He was afraid of losing himself to her control. He feared that he would become just a product of her caretaking efforts. In his business, and on the golf course, he could be his own man.

So Darla had to back off. She had to let him be the way he wanted to be. She had to renounce her control of him. That was the only way he would ever feel secure enough to open up to her again. That might never happen—it hasn't happened yet—but it's also the only way she could get on with her own life.

4. Pick your battles. This is one of those extremely practical points that must be added to this pile of psychological advice. It sounds good to let go and renounce control, but what happens in the trenches when Johnny needs new shoes and your mate has just spent your last dollar on a new nine-iron?

In the gritty day-to-day of life, you're going to need to decide some things together. There will be conflicts. You will need to control some things for the survival of your family or yourself.

So pick your battles. Don't make a federal case out of every disagreement. Let a lot of stuff slide. But when there's an issue that your spouse must address—when his or her behavior has to change—address it. Make your case as best as you can.

If you're haggling over every detail, that will create a war-like atmosphere, and it will draw you further into the downward spiral. But if you choose your battles carefully, you can accomplish most of what you need to, while staying free of over-entanglement.

5. Find your own identity. Psychologists have noted that security and significance are basic factors of every person's identity. When these are shaken, our lives are in turmoil.

It's natural for us to find these in our spouses. There's a sense of emotional security in knowing "I will always be loved by this person" or at least a practical security in knowing "I have someone to be with." We can find significance in the thought that "I am important to this person" or "I affect this person's life in a major way."

The process of detaching involves finding your security and significance apart from your relationship with your spouse. Who are you—on your own? How would you manage by yourself? What good are you without a spouse to care for? These are hard questions, but you must ask them.

Please understand that this is not my typical marital advice. For most couples, security and significance are found in their marriage relationship. And that's the way I believe it should be. But what are Darla and other women like her to do when they get little or no affirmation from their spouses?

As I've said, I work regularly with people who are newly divorced. Many of them are literally in a daze. The rug has been pulled out from under them. Their most basic sense of security and significance is shaken. I remember that feeling from when my first wife left me. I didn't know who I was.

Detachment within a marriage takes you through that process more slowly to shore yourself up against the impending storm. As you consider these basic questions, and find new answers, you will lessen your unhealthy dependence on your spouse.

Try this. Get a sheet of paper and write down ten answers to the question: "Who are you?" You might include talents, temperaments, interests, relationships, faith, opinions, background, work, and so on. Now go back through that list and cross out everything directly related to your spouse. If you needed to be totally on your own, would these things apply?

You're probably left with eight or nine things that describe you. *You.* Just you. Not as wife of So-and-so or husband of What's-her-name. This could be the beginning of an awareness of your own self. You can think in the singular case now. You can develop your individual identity.

Consider questions like this:

- What is your political persuasion: Do you favor Democrats, Republicans, or independents?
- What is your favorite TV show or movie or play?
- What is the best feature of your personality?
- If you received $300,000 in the mail today, what would you do with it?
- When have you felt closest to God?
- If you had a year to travel, where would you go?
- What do you think is the greatest need of our country today?

Obviously, these are just starter questions. But if you can answer them for yourself, without checking your spouse's opinion, that's good. This may seem very basic, but remember our case study with Sally? She was in an unhealthy marriage for seventeen years. Her husband gradually chipped away at her self-esteem, to the point where she had no opinions of her own. She didn't know she could have a favorite TV show. If you gave her $300,000, she'd give it to her husband to handle.

Detachment involves finding yourself, getting to know who you are.

6. Find something to do. This can shore up your sense of significance. Get a job if you don't have one. Volunteer for a church or charitable organization. Take up an artistic pursuit or hobby.

Darla finished her degree and got a job. That was an attempt at detachment. Stan accepted this, largely because they could use the money, but he had some resentment, too. This is not uncommon. As you begin to establish your own identity and activities, your spouse may feel threatened. You are beginning to break free, and that puts the relationship on unfamiliar turf. But stay with it. You need to realize that you can have some significance outside the marital relationship.

7. Develop new friendships. Friends can give you emotional security. If all else falls apart, they will be there for you. Friends also encourage you in the difficult times—and, as you know, there are many difficult times. Friends can critique you as well. If your judgment is faulty, if your plans are foolish, if your attitudes are out of line, good friends will tell you so (especially if you give them permission).

As I've said earlier in this book, addictive relationships have a way of folding in on themselves. The partners focus on each other and let other friendships slide. Often, one jealous partner will discourage or forbid the other from having outside friendships. Part of this process of finding yourself involves finding your own friends.

Darla did this. As she got increasingly frustrated with Stan, she turned to friends at work and church for emotional support. This was an important part of her own return to health. She cautions, however, that it's important to find friends who understand your goals. Several people she began to confide in were quick to say, "Dump him!" They didn't understand her commitment to the marriage. She needed people to help her through this difficult process of becoming a whole person while staying in the marriage.

8. Become self-sufficient in some practical matters. A friend told me about his grandmother, who lost her husband when they were both about sixty. For forty years, she relied on him for the practical matters of running the home. She took care of the inside of the home—cooking and cleaning—but he wrote the checks, ran the errands, and paid the bills. After his death, she was at a loss. She couldn't get a credit card. She had a hard time dealing with the insurance company. She had to learn to drive all over again.

Many women are like that today—totally dependent on their husbands for any financial matters. This isn't necessarily bad, but if there's a general pattern of unhealthy dependency, this can add to it. Many men, too, are at a loss when it comes to the upkeep of the home, raising children, or cooking. (Forgive me for perpetuating the sexual stereotypes, but many homes still adopt these traditional roles.)

It would help you to learn some of these practical matters. If you were suddenly single, what would you need to know to function on your own? In Darla's case, she got a job and began to make a modest living of her own, so she wouldn't be dependent on Stan's rising and falling business interests.

You may be thinking, *Preparing for divorce. That's all this is.* Believe me, that's not my intention. But it is all a part of detachment. When one partner is unhealthily dependent on the other, those dependencies need to be changed. In the ways I've just listed, you may be able to let go of some things that are messing up the relationship and find yourself. The ideal is that you and your partner might eventually come together on different and more healthy terms. A great amount of healing and change will have to take place first, but there's always hope.

If you have chosen this heroic route, I commend your choice. You have not chosen the seemingly easier route—to start over with someone else. Instead, you have chosen to honor your commitment in marriage. I hope that you'll be able to find yourself, and then to rediscover a new, healthier marriage.

Chapter Seventeen

Addiction in a Same-sex Friendship

֍

CARA AND KIM ARE BOTH TWENTY-FIVE YEARS OLD. THEY BECAME FAST friends in high school and have talked to each other at least once a day ever since. Both have boyfriends, and they often double-date. Even when they don't double, they regularly compare notes about their dates.

At one point a few years ago, Kim struck up a friendship with a new secretary, Betty, in the office where she worked. They would often take lunch breaks together. Every so often she would mention to Cara that "Betty said this" or "Betty did that." Cara became quite jealous, though she wouldn't admit it at first, even to herself. But she feared that Betty was taking her place as Kim's best friend, and she didn't know how she would survive without that friendship.

Subtly at first, but then more openly, Cara signaled her disapproval of Kim's new friend. She began to change her schedule to have lunch with Kim more often, and she warned Kim that Betty might be "using" her to get in good with people at the office. Kim eventually cut back on her lunches with Betty, but Cara still seemed paranoid about that friendship. Ultimately, Cara found a new job for Kim, near where she herself worked.

Kim was concerned about the jealousy shown by Cara, but she enjoyed Cara's friendship and didn't want to threaten it. Earlier this year, Kim took an impulsive weekend trip to New England with her boyfriend. When she returned, Cara was furious.

"You didn't tell me a thing about this," Cara charged. "I called you all weekend. I thought you died or something. I was worried sick."

Even when Kim explained how sudden it all was, Cara scolded her for not letting her help plan the weekend, and for not inviting Cara and her boyfriend along.

This made Kim feel guilty. She apologized profusely and bent over backwards in the next few weeks to be a good friend to Cara.

A New Environment for Addiction

Though this book has focused primarily on romantic relationships, I've also mentioned other environments for addictive relationships. Cara and Kim clearly show symptoms of an addictive relationship, and we can transfer many of the same principles from romances to same-sex friendships.

Kim and Cara aren't lesbians. There's no sexual or romantic involvement here. It is true that some homosexuals develop this kind of emotional dependency, but it doesn't necessarily indicate that the friends are gay. (Certainly, many other issues are involved in homosexual relationships. I won't address them specifically here.)

Emotional dependency is more common in female friendships, but not exclusive to them. I once had a male friend who sort of attached himself to me and grew too dependent on our friendship. He was not gay, just emotionally dependent, but it was an unhealthy situation and I had to ease out of it. Still, in our culture, the deepest emotional bonding seems to occur among women. (It's also possible for male-female friendships to develop an emotional dependency without being romantic, but that's rare.)

Defining the Problem

Where do you draw the line? Where does a good friendship go bad? Is it wrong to call a friend every day? Is it wrong to compare notes about your love life?

Go back to chapter 4 to check out the characteristics of unhealthy addictive relationships. Those same principles apply. In the case of Kim and Cara, we see a friendship that's definitely out of balance.

We see it first in the exclusive nature of the friendship. It's a closed circle—no one else can get in. Even the boyfriends are on the outskirts, it seems. When the exclusivity is breached, jealousy rears its ugly head. Powerful negative feelings arise, even if they're irrational.

In a healthy friendship, Cara would rejoice with Kim in her discovery of a new friend. She might try to befriend Betty herself, suggesting that the three of them go out together. Healthy relationships are inclusive. The more the merrier.

Hidden beneath the jealousy is a lack of trust. Cara does not trust that Kim will continue to be a friend to her if she has other friends, or if she goes off with her boyfriend somewhere—outside of Cara's control. This lack of trust often comes from poor self-esteem. If I don't believe that I am worth befriending, I'm afraid that you will run off to a better friend.

That poor self-esteem also shows up in a lack of boundaries. As I said in chapter 15, good fences make good partners. Good fences also make good friends. I need to know where I end and where you begin. What are my responsibilities and what are yours? What privacy do I have? What decisions can I make by myself?

Whatever boundaries Kim may have had, Cara crossed. Kim could not go off with her boyfriend without asking Cara to help plan it, and maybe to go along! Kim could not make other friends. And Cara even found Kim a new job, exercising her control in that way, too. It's as if Cara needed to live Kim's life for her.

So far, I'm making Cara seem like a real villain. But Kim is a willing accomplice. I recognize some aspects of a caretaker in Kim. She sees that Cara needs her, and she responds to that. (Note that the new secretary needed a friend in her new office, and Kim rushed to help her, too.)

She's not as directly dependent on Cara as Cara is on her, but she responds to Cara's dependency. Cara lays a guilt trip on her, and Kim feels guilty.

Cara, in effect, says, "I needed you and you weren't there for me."

How does Kim respond? She could say, "That's not true. I've always been there for you, but your demands are unreasonable. I needed to get away."

But no. She says, "You're right. I'm sorry. It won't happen again." She allows Cara to erase the boundaries between them. Apparently Kim has certain needs that get met when she gives in to Cara. She feels responsible for Cara's well-being, and so she allows Cara to invade her life. If she didn't do this, she would be a bad person—or so she thinks.

Both would be healthier if they could put up some boundaries. Cara needs to get a life of her own and to be happy with that. The best thing Kim could do for Cara is to withdraw and to force Cara into some self-sufficiency.

How to Find Healing

How will these two achieve a healthy friendship? Maybe they can't. They may be in too deep. If you've read the rest of this book, it won't surprise you that if the relationship is far out of balance then I recommend a complete cold-turkey separation. As with any addiction, moderation is not an effective strategy. The best thing for Cara and Kim would be to withdraw from each other for at least a year. It would be hard to do, and painful, but it's the best way.

If that's impossible, then a backup strategy would be something like what I suggest for those in addictive marriages: detachment. If you must keep some sort of friendship in place, at least put some distance between you. Set up some boundaries, make some rules.

With Kim and Cara, I might suggest that they limit their phone calls to once or twice a week, rather than every day.

It might also be healthy to stay away from conversation about their boyfriends. (This might be unnecessary, but I suspect that those romantic relationships may be stunted by the constant interaction between the two friends.)

Further, I would urge both friends to be sensitive about guilt-mongering. Cara should try to recognize when she is laying a guilt trip on Kim, and avoid doing it. Kim should recognize that, too, and refuse to buckle under.

I'd also recommend that both friends get involved in some new activity that they keep private from the other. This would allow each person to grow individually, apart from the other person's control.

Such measures may or may not get the friendship on a healthier course. If the dependency is mild, this may be the way to go. The friendship could continue on healthier terms. But if there's a serious emotional addiction, I still recommend a complete break. I know that sounds harsh: splitting up best friends. But in cases like that, the relationship has grown beyond friendship into an unhealthy attachment.

Besides distancing themselves from each other, Kim and Cara need to take a serious look at why the relationship got so far out of balance in the first place. Their relationship is just a symptom of a deeper problem. Even if they distance themselves from each other, they're only treating the symptom. Each will probably replace that missing friendship with a new relationship with someone else. More specifically, I would suspect that their boyfriends would soon replace that missing need, and a romantic addiction could easily develop. Therefore, it's essential that any correction of an addictive relationship be accompanied by a commitment to address the issues that led to the problem.

When a friendship is healthy, it becomes a resource for personal growth. For those prone to addictive relationships, friendships are essential for accountability, they provide affirmation and support, they help people to learn trust and unconditional love, and they become a springboard for all other relationships.

In chapter 4, I contrasted characteristics of healthy relationships with those of addictive relationships. Let me review some of those as they apply specifically in a friendship.

1. Friends get together because they enjoy each other's company, not because they feel any compulsive need or guilt when they don't see each other.
2. Friendships are mutual and reciprocal. They are not driven by a need to rescue, but instead contain elements of mutually helping each other through support and encouragement.
3. Friendships are honest and objective. People can feel free to share their feelings with their friends, knowing they won't be judged. They also know their friends will give them objective feedback, not tainted with an overly negative perspective or blinded by rose-colored glasses.
4. Friendships are inclusive. Sure, there are times when you want to be alone with your best friend, but generally, good friends enjoy the company of other friends.
5. Friends trust each other. They aren't jealous when they hear about your other friends.
6. Friends are whole people who enjoy each other but aren't dependent on each other.
7. Friends build each other up. Their relationship is growing and supportive. They do not punish, shame, or in any way weaken the other person. Their relationship is not a love-hate cycle, but rather a slow, steady, growing friendship.

CHAPTER EIGHTEEN

Family Relationships

ℰↄ

EVEN IN FAMILY SETTINGS, THE MOST BASIC OF HUMAN RELATIONSHIPS, healthy attachments can become unhealthy. True love can become emotional dependency. And it can go both ways: a parent dependent on children or a child clinging too long to parents. We'll talk first about a parent's overattachment to a child.

Parent-child Dependency

At the beginning of life, there are no boundaries between a mother and child. The child is physically part of the mother's body, wholly dependent. After the birth, the baby remains dependent, though obviously less attached in a physical way. Both father and mother care for the child—feeding it, clothing it, and making virtually all of its decisions. As the child grows, it develops a will of its own. Every parent knows that the child's will does not always conform to the parents' will. But in most cases, the parent stays in control up to the teen years, when the child assumes more and more responsibility for him or herself. A problem occurs when parents fail to let go, trying to maintain control of their children's lives well into adulthood. That control needs to be released.

The goal of parenting is to create independent, healthy individuals. It's a give-and-take process that encourages the growth, decision-making, and independent thinking of the child. Obviously, some measures of independence that would be fine for a seventeen-year-old would be inappropriate for a twelve-year-old. But healthy child-rearing always moves in the direction of independence. *Good parents are always preparing to let go.*

When a parent continues to "baby" a child, something's wrong. Parents who make decisions for an adult child or impose opinions on every aspect of the adult child's life are not letting go. If a parent is unable to accept the independence of a grown child, there's an unhealthy addiction at work.

In a lecture based on his book *The Road Less Traveled*, M. Scott Peck observed an interesting paradox: "Children who grew up in warm, nurturing, loving homes usually had relatively little difficulty in leaving those homes. Whereas children who grew up in homes filled with backbiting, hostility, coldness, and viciousness, often had a great deal of trouble leaving such homes."[1]

Dr. Peck goes on to point out that this observation, while illogical, is nonetheless a reflection of the fact that children from dysfunctional families become enmeshed in the dysfunctional system and then view the world as a hostile, uncaring place. Parents who raise their children in a healthy environment teach them independence and what he calls "separateness." As they grow up, the children look forward to the challenges of the outside world, and are much better prepared to face that world. He concludes by saying, "Ultimately, it is the goal of the parent to help the child separate."

A Case in Point

Remember Bonnie? She had a bad trip to the mission field with a scoundrel of a husband, and she's had several bad romances since. But as she tells of her troubles, she keeps referring to her parents' opinions. Whether she admits it or not, she is controlled by them, though she is well into her thirties.

Her parents continue to pass judgment on her decisions. And Bonnie, with that childhood longing for Daddy's approval, lets those judgments affect her decisions. She complains that they "baby" her, that they're holding her back from reaching her potential, and yet she is irrationally drawn back to them. She lacks the strength to defy their opinions.

It's interesting to see how these things get passed from one generation to the next. Bonnie has a teenage daughter who's considering going off to college. Bonnie is emotionally devastated by this prospect and is doing all she can to make sure the daughter stays home. "It's not safe," she tells her daughter. "Wait until you're older. You'll get lonely being so far from home." The truth is, Bonnie fears her own loneliness, her own lack of safety. She finds a certain security in her attachment to her daughter, and she can't let go.

We often see this happening among mothers whose children are leaving the nest. Our culture (at least part of our traditional culture) has conveyed the message that a woman's sole value is in motherhood. When the children are no longer around to mother, there's a major identity crisis. A mother can lose her sense of significance. What does she do now? Some just try to keep mothering their children—to an unhealthy point.

The tendency is less severe among fathers, who often find their significance elsewhere. But they sometimes experience a crisis of control. A father of grown children can be like the corporate president whose company goes bankrupt—he's not in charge of anything anymore. All he can do is to be a consultant.

A single friend of mine joked that whenever she visits her parents, her mom gives her food and her dad gives her advice. "Without fail," she said. "It happens every time."

This isn't necessarily unhealthy. But these trends can reach a point where they indicate an unhealthy addiction to one's children. How do you know when it's a problem?

Symptoms

When parents seek to control the life of their grown child, it's dangerous. It's one thing to give advice. It's another to get upset when the advice is not followed. It's even worse to apply emotional, financial or practical pressure to ensure that the advice is followed. Like spouses, parents often know the emotional buttons to push to get their way.

Also watch for role reversals. If a parent gets too emotionally dependent, the child may actually take on a parental role. The child is forced to make decisions about the relationship: "Yes, you may go shopping with me"; "No, I don't have time to talk now." In order to maintain his or her own health, the child is forced to determine the bounds of the relationship.

And that's another danger sign: boundary violations. Parents sometimes get too enmeshed in their children's lives. They have to know everything the child is doing, and some need to be involved in it all, too. They may invade their children's privacy in other ways. They may identify with their children too much, living life vicariously through them. As with any other relationship, they need to build healthy boundaries: that's your life, this is mine.

Restoration

How do you restore these relationships? In most cases, I'd treat these like addictive marriages: Cold turkey is not the best way to go. If you can redefine the relationship on healthier terms, do it.

If you're a parent and you find yourself unhealthily enmeshed with your child's life, you need to learn to let go. This may involve a certain mental reorientation. You need to enjoy the independence of your children. Remember, that's the goal of parenting. Recognize your attempts to cling to your children, and try to talk yourself into letting go. Your children will make some mistakes. You cannot spare them the pain of those mistakes. It is only through such mistakes that they learn.

I heard a story about the mother of a physically disabled child who was talking with a friend. The child was playing nearby and he fell—not seriously. The mother looked on as the boy struggled to get back up. With his disability, it wasn't easy, but eventually the boy was back on his feet.

The friend was astonished. "Why didn't you help him?" she asked the mother.

"I did," the mother replied.

It takes the wisdom of Solomon to know when to step in and when to back off. Parents have a difficult task. But if you're aware of an unhealthy attachment with your child, learn the wisdom of that disabled boy's mother. You help the most by letting your child do it himself.

Decide on boundaries and observe them. Discuss these with your child, or just adopt them yourself. You might limit the time spent with your child or on the phone. You might limit the advice you give or even the financial aid you offer.

Learn your child's emotional "hot buttons" and stay away. As a parent, you can destroy your kid with a word. You have that power. You know instinctively how to cut to the core of that person. Part of healthy boundary-observing is to train your instincts to stay away from sore spots. Talk with your child about what these are.

Get a life. As you develop your own skills, interests, and personality—outside of parenting—you will have less of a need to invade your child's life.

Strategies for the Adult Child

What do you do if you are the grown child of a parent who won't let go?

Talk about it. Tell your parent(s) of your need for independence. Work through the steps listed above, especially boundary-setting.

Sidestep the guilt trip. If your parents don't understand your needs, they may do all they can to instill guilt. Don't buy it. You are trying to save a relationship—just as a spouse might work to save a marriage. You are merely recognizing that the current state of affairs is not healthy. You are trying to establish the ground rules for a new, healthy relationship. You are actually trying to help them do a better job of parenting you. It may seem selfish, but in the long run it's the best thing for them as well.

Detach if necessary. If your parents refuse to abide by proper boundaries, you may need to distance yourself. Move away or stay away for a time. Or even if you must maintain some contact, limit the ways in which you cooperate with their control of you. You don't have to tell them everything. You don't have to seek or accept their advice. The goal is always to come back together at some future point in a more healthy way. But even if that doesn't happen, all the individuals involved need to find their own emotional health.

Child-parent Dependencies

Reverse the fields. Let's talk about when a child won't let go of his or her parents. This is especially problematic as it affects one's marriage.

Rick and Nancy came to me for counseling. "Nancy sees or calls her mother every day," Rick complained.

What's wrong with that?" Nancy replied.

"But it's all the time," Rick explained. "She'll call her from work. Then she'll stop by on the way home from work. Then she'll call her after dinner and chat for an hour or more. I sometimes think her mother is more important to her than I am."

"That's ridiculous," Nancy said, rolling her eyes.

Rick went on. "About six months ago, Nan got a promotion at work. Great news, right? She comes home, says, 'Hi, hon,' and heads right for the phone. I overhear her telling her mother about her promotion. That's how I found out about it."

Nancy was shaking her head. "You don't understand."

"It seems like any decision we make has to be approved by her mother," Rick added. "We can't just decide to go on vacation. We have to check Mom for the dates and destination."

"She'd been to Cape Cod and didn't like it, that's all" Nancy explained. "She said it was better in the fall."

But Rick was on a roll. "The worst of it is when her mother gets me on the phone and says personal stuff that Nancy hasn't even talked with me about."

"Like what?" Nancy challenged.

"Like, 'So, Rick, Nancy says you haven't been very energetic in bed lately. What's wrong? You working too hard?' "

"She did not say that!"

"She most certainly did!"

You get the idea. A week before I saw them, they had an awful fight (imagine that!) and she walked out.

Guess where she went? Mother's.

In private counseling a week later, Nancy told me that, if she had to choose between Rick and her mother, she'd choose Mom. "After all, I've only known him four years and I've known her all my life."

Evaluation

In my opinion, Nancy has an unhealthy, perhaps addictive, relationship with her mother. There's a lack of independence in decision-making and obvious violation of personal and marital boundaries. In addition, the relationship seems to be rather exclusive in shutting out Nancy's own husband.

The biblical book of Genesis offers some ancient wisdom on the subject. Adam calls Eve "bone of my bone and flesh of my flesh" and the writer adds the comment: "For this reason a man will leave his father and mother and be united to his wife, and they will become one flesh."[2]

For both men and women, leaving parents is an important step toward good marriages and other healthy relationships. It doesn't mean you never talk to them or you disdain what they say. But your priorities change. You develop new loyalties.

Nancy, and the many people like her, need to adopt the same strategies we have been talking about—detachment and boundaries. With proper communication, joint effort, and a firm decision to change, the unhealthy parent-child relationship can turn into a healthy friendship with appropriate limits.

CHAPTER NINETEEN

Conclusion

❦

IN THIS BOOK, YOU'VE MET A NUMBER OF PEOPLE, ALL OF WHOM struggled with unhealthy relationships that would be considered addictive in some way. Sally, Christine, Scott, and the others had unique situations, but I'm sure you've recognized some common threads throughout.

That was the secret of the original circle I convened in chapter 1. Each member had his or her own story, but they had similar sufferings. Each person could say to the others, "I know what you're going through or I don't know exactly what you're going through, but I've felt something like it."

The problem with a book like this is that I don't know exactly what you're going through. I don't know why you picked up this book. I have no idea of the impact it will have in your life. Your situation is unique.

And yet you can learn from Sally, Christine, and the others. Their stories and the principles presented here may help you cope with your particular problems. It's up to you, though, to sift through them—to toss out what doesn't apply and cling to what does. It's up to you.

It's always tempting to sit back and let a book do your

healing for you. After all, you've done your job—reading it—now it's time for your miracle cure, right?

It doesn't work like that. Now is the time for you to get to work, putting this book's ideas into practice. It will take discipline on your part and some tough decisions. Maybe you'll need to say no to an old lover or yes to some new friends. Maybe you'll need to climb out of self-pity and join a bowling team or a theater group. Maybe you need to get more serious about your work or about the friends who have quietly been supporting you through this whole thing.

The God Factor

Maybe you need to get more serious about God and how you view His role in your process of changing and healing.

In this regard, there are two kinds of people reading this book. I'm tempted to call them "religious" and "not religious," but that's not exactly it. And it's not just a matter of believing in God or not. It's more a matter of living by faith.

You see, some people depend on God in their day-to-day lives. He's a guide, a teacher, a comforter. These people have been reading this book wondering when we're going to get around to the "main point"—the miracles God is going to work to cure you of your love problems.

Maybe you're one of these people. Or maybe not. There are many who prefer to work out their own problems. If you sit around expecting a miracle, they figure, you'll probably just sit around. In this life, you make your own miracles.

Well, you're both right.

I do believe that God heals people. Sometimes He defies all medical expectations and works a miracle. But I still see a doctor when I'm sick because I believe that God regularly uses natural processes of healing, and doctors are trained to recognize and enhance those natural processes.

The same holds true for emotional healing. There are natural processes by which people are healed. Detachment. Renewed identity and self-esteem. Balance and boundaries. All of these can help people break free from unhealthy dependencies. To say "Just trust in God and He will make it all better" is to ignore the processes by which He makes it better.

Yet I do believe in miracles. I sincerely thought Sally would die from her addictions, but here she is in front of me—happy, confident, and free. That's a miracle.

Laurie was in the pits of despair over her failed relationship with her boss. She talks about learning to depend on God. She praises God for bringing her back to health. That, too, is a miracle.

Twelve-step programs, starting with Alcoholics Anonymous, have recognized the need to depend on a Higher Power. Part of the healing process is to come to the end of your own strength and to reach out for divine aid. I've seen that happen in case after case after case.

Churches spend a lot of effort trying to help people become holy. Unfortunately, holiness has taken on some bad connotations. In popular imagery, a holy person is one who has no fun and doesn't want anyone else to have fun. But linguistically, "holiness" is essentially the same as "wholeness." Yes, God wants to make us holy. He also wants to make us whole.

If you are feeling partial these days, if a chunk of you is missing, if you seem to have lost that part of you that makes good decisions or enjoys healthy relationships, if you are craving the love you never got as a child, or if you are desperately reaching for some mystery ingredient that our society keeps saying you need, God can make you whole. Having a relationship with this Higher Power is a matter of surrendering your life to Him, trusting that He knows what is best for your life. He's the only one who can fill the void of an empty life. No relationship, no lover, and certainly no addiction can do that.

Miracles happen, even today. Recovery is possible in your life, but miracles usually happen to moving targets.

After reading this book, you know what you need to do. Now do it. Your miracle could begin today. Maybe it has already begun.

Notes

ℊ

Chapter One: The Circle
1. Gerald G. May, *Addiction and Grace* (San Francisco: Harper, 1988), p. 13.

Chapter Two: Types of Addictive Relationships
1. Robert Palmer, "Addicted to Love." Copyright © 1985, Bungalow Music, NY. Used by permission. All rights reserved.
2. Genesis 2:24.
3. Computing Magazine, June/July issue, John C. Dvorak, "Net Addiction" WWW. PCCOWUTING.COK June/July 1996, p. 85.

Chapter Four: Characteristics of Addictive Relationships
1. Howard Halpern, *How to Break Your Addiction to a Person* (New York: Bantam, 1982), pp. 7–8.
2. M. Scott Peck, *The Road Less Traveled* (New York: Simon and Schuster, 1978), p. 91.
3. M. Scott Peck, *The Road Less Traveled*, p. 92.

Chapter Seven: The Roots of Addiction
1. Daniel Goleman, "Drug Addiction Linked to Brain Chemistry," Santa Barbara News Press, July 7, 1990.
2. Carolyn Johnson, *Understanding Alcoholism* (Grand Rapids: Zondervan, 1991), pp. 28–29.
3. Archibald Hart, *Healing Life's Hidden Addictions* (Ann Arbor: Servant, 1990), pp. 44–53.

Chapter Sixteen: Addiction Within a Marriage
1. Gerald G. May, *Addiction and Grace*, p. 3.
2. M. Scott Peck, "Further Along the Road Less Traveled," lecture, 1988.

Chapter Eighteen: Family Relationships
1. M. Scott Peck, "Further Along the Road Less Traveled," lecture, 1988.
2. Genesis 2:24.

About the Authors

℘

DR. THOMAS WHITEMAN is the founder and president of Life Counseling Services with offices throughout Eastern Pennsylvania and New Jersey. He's also the coauthor of numerous books, including the *Fresh Start Divorce Recovery Workbook, Adult ADD, The Marriage Mender*, and *The Complete Stress Management Workbook*. He and his wife, Lori, have three children, Elizabeth, Michelle, and Kurt.

Randy Petersen has written more than twenty books, including several with Thomas Whiteman on psychology and self-help themes and small-group curriculum for youth and adults. He's also involved in theater as a director, actor, acting teacher, and playwright.

For more information on seminars, counseling services, and other resources, contact:

Life Counseling Services
63 Chestnut Rd.
Paoli, PA 19301
1-800-882-2799

WHO'S TO BLAME?

If you're tired of being hurt by the hurting
people in your life, this book will give you
the handle you need on the dynamics
of victimization and blame.

Who's to Blame?

(Carmen Renee Berry & Mark W. Baker) $14

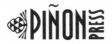